P.

# Women Only

"Moving and heartfelt. Dr. Birken expresses the physician's side of the patient relationship with grace and candor."
**Craig A. Miller, M.D.**, author,
*The Making of a Surgeon in the 21st Century*

"Dr. Birken is authentic, empathetic, and utterly human in his amalgam of 'tales' on those conditions that most impact women's lives. His 'creative non-fiction' will intrigue, and lighten, and inspire readers of both genders."
**James A. Schaller, M.D.**, author,
*Do Yourself a Favor: Love Your Wife*

"Dr. Randy Birken writes the stories of these women as if he has known them all his life—in reality he did. The relationship between a gynecologist and a patient transcends all what is not modern medicine. It is more than the framework of the business—it is sometimes more about the trust."
**Sharon Messimer**, Marketing Director
for Memorial Hermann Healthcare System

"Randy Birken, M.D., writes with insight and compassion about the many health issues of concern to women and he gives those issues appealing human faces, inspiring readers to share in the sorrows and joys, seriousness and humor that are a part of every woman's life."
**Rosemary Poole-Carter**, published novelist and playwright

"Dr. Birken's clinical vignettes bring gynecologic medicine to life in a readable, entertaining, and medically accurate series of 'glimpses' into the lives of women. What an enjoyable way to learn!"
**Dorothy Roach, M.D.**, Director, North Houston
Center for Reproductive Medicine.

"Dr. Birken does a superb job in bringing human warmth and humor to an otherwise, clinical profession. His unique approach to revealing the strength and composure of his patients in crisis allows the reader to enter the inner world of doctor and patient, a heretofore revered and confidential one, to become a part of the story. Dr. Birken is a renowned doctor in his own right, but had the courage to seek additional training in the art of creative writing, having obtained a Master of Liberal Arts Degree in Literature twenty years after his M.D. His patient-composite approach is refreshing and avoids many of the pitfalls that occur in other medical accounts of the doctor-patient relationship that usually come across as clinical and perfunctory. His chronological approach, using the woman's lifespan as a guidepost to the myriad of illnesses awaiting an otherwise healthy female medically and psychologically, is both intriguing and inspirational. Dr. Birken has a potential bestseller, and women and men will buy this book if they want an inside look at the ideal doctor-patient relationship at a time when patient trust in organized medicine is lacking. Those who enjoyed Oliver Sacks' *The Man Who Mistook his Wife for a Hat*, will find Dr. Birken's book an equally seminal one on doctoring with humility, humor, and humanness."

**A. Keith Barton, Ph.D.**, psychologist and published author

"The title of this work, *Women Only*, may be a bit misleading and that would indeed be unfortunate. Though the subjects are women, the message is one that should be of relevance to fathers, husbands and especially daughters. Dr. Birken has done an excellent job of translating clinical and case study data into words that can be readily understood by the lay person. With care and sensitivity he explains and deals with both physical and emotional issues that most women, at some developmental stage, will no doubt confront. Dr. Birken is obviously not only an able clinician, but an excellent teller of important and helpful stories."

**David Gottlieb, Ph.D.**, former Dean of the College of Social Sciences at the University of Houston and published author

# Women Only

## The Gynecologist Is In:
## Real Life Stories

## RANDY A. BIRKEN, M.D.

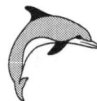

BLUE DOLPHIN PUBLISHING

Published by Blue Dolphin Publishing, Inc.
P.O. Box 8, Nevada City, CA 95959
Orders: 1-800-643-0765
Web: www.bluedolphinpublishing.com

ISBN: 978-1-57733-225-1  paperback
ISBN: 978-1-57733-252-7  hardcover


Library of Congress Cataloging-in-Publication Data

Birken, Randy A., 1950-
    Women only : the gynecologist is in : real life stories / Randy
A. Birken.
        p. cm.
    ISBN 978-1-57733-252-7 (hardcover : alk. paper) —
ISBN 978-1-57733-225-1 (pbk. : alk. paper)
    1. Gynecology—Popular works. I. Title.
    RG121.B457 2010
    618.1—dc22
                                                                2010002529

Printed in the United States of America

10    9    8    7    6    5    4    3    2    1

# Table of Contents

# PART I

# Introduction

CHAPTER 1

# Doctoring and the Human Experience

WOMEN'S HEALTH AND ILLNESS is a complex subject involving the disciplines of physical, physiological, and pathological states. The issues influencing gynecological care enhance or even transcend basic medical sciences—social, cultural, and, most importantly, psychological factors—which create unique and individual perceptions of health and disease.

Women can obtain medical information, and the associated social impact on their lives, from many sources: the Internet, magazines, TV, radio, word-of-mouth, as well as healthcare providers. Yet these sources are limited to specifics and are void of the "human" shape of health and illness. What form of information can bridge these compromises and provide an overall depiction of the human dimension or the human experience? Answer: The "case study"—clinical stories about individuals enduring disease or diseases, and the ramifications on their lives.

Perhaps Drs. Richard Reynolds and John Stone define this concept best in their book, *On Doctoring*:

> In the process of caring for their patients, physicians have a unique— and privileged—window on the full range of human emotions. Literature, too, is rich in its descriptions of individual illnesses and plagues, in its capacity to reveal patients' reactions to illnesses, and doctors' dilemmas in providing care.

But why the "case study," a narrative of a person's medical problem or problems? Dr. Oliver Sacks, in his compelling book, *The Man Who Mistook His Wife for a Hat and Other Clinical Tales*,

3

presents neurological "case studies" in a way that is insightful as well as fascinating. Is it the intrigue of being a "fly on the wall," or the identification of a character that "feels" real when compared to plain facts and figures? Or is it the added ingredient of physician/patient psychodynamics, as well as the frailties and emotional reactions of doctors? Laura Miller, in her article entitled "Scheherazade in the Consulting Room," appearing in the *Sunday New York Times Book Review* on June 15, 2003, believes that it is both:

> Yet it's just this little chink, through which the wayward reality of a human being escapes, eluding even the most gifted doctor, that lends the finishing touch of verisimilitude. It's the most satisfying twist of all.

Not only does the non-medical reader benefit and learn from the case study, but physicians and medical students as well. While teaching "Medicine, Literature, and the Human Condition" at Baylor College of Medicine, this author noticed that students responded positively to the inspiring readings and left the conference room with a more energized spirit and a renewed commitment to the medical profession. The overwhelming technological overload the students face day-in-and-day-out throughout their medical education is softened by the compassion and tenderness of case studies that are humanistic and heart-warming.

Studying literary works with medical themes exposes these intelligent individuals to the perspective of the patient, hence promoting compassion and greater empathy, while the topic of medical ethics promotes professional integrity and responsibility. Additionally, these literary works provide a catharsis for students who are burdened with the complexities of medical science as well as medical liability, consumerism, and managed health care. But most importantly, students learn to refocus their reasons for becoming doctors—the nobility of the profession—emphasizing the practice of medicine as an art as well as a science.

These case histories work just as well for physicians already in practice, creating a revived commitment to care-giving often mitigated by the constraints of managed health care and medical-legal pressures. In an article from the medical journal, *Lancet*, entitled, "Why literature and medicine?" Drs. McLellan and Jones emphasize the importance of incorporating literature into medical school curriculums and for the value of its exposure to practicing physicians:

> Some outcomes of learning to read this way—a way that focuses on literary analysis of complex texts—are thought to be increased empathetic understanding, development of complex interpretive skills, and a greater appreciation for the art of medicine by students and practitioners.

Therefore, with this definition for teaching literary works with medical themes and the role of the case study, what is the purpose for this collection of clinical stories? For the same reasons that apply to medical students and physicians, this concept is appropriate for a non-medical audience—to inform, to enlighten, to inspire the human spirit—a spirit that is universal and transcends social, cultural, racial, religious, as well as gender differences.

While some stories in this collection are warm and tender, others are emotionally visceral and present a tragic commentary on human frailties and social conditions. Topics that extend throughout the life span of a woman—the unusual but delicate pediatric conditions; adolescent problems such as eating disorders, drug and alcohol abuse, and the complexities of parental interaction; young adult issues including the confusion of new responsibilities, sexually transmitted diseases, adoption and abortion; the emotional consequences of infertility and obstetrical problems; surgical complications and its repercussions; domestic violence and divorce; the physical and emotional distress of obesity; mid-life to older age issues, including menopause, cancer, and the loss of a spouse; and the human side of physicians: their feelings, their lives as doctors, and their interaction with patients and other physicians.

Although these "tales" deal with women and their associated problems, every male knows a female intimately, either as spouse, partner, mother, sister, aunt, niece, cousin, or friend, which brings them into the arena of women's health. That which affects someone we love affects us as well.

It must be emphasized that these stories are composites of many experiences and not of a single patient's medical life. This style of writing serves many purposes: to protect the confidentiality of the patient, a most important and "sacred" part of medical practice—and to present an amalgam of health issues in an intriguing and inspiring way, while incorporating as many different topics as possible. This "creative non-fiction" is not intended to deceive or dupe the reader, but to enhance the edification derived from the readings. For this author, writing to enlighten is as satisfying as providing the most conscientious and compassionate care to patients—a reward that compensates for all the hours of hard work, and all the burdens of a most demanding profession.

PART II

# The Pre-adolescent Years

# CHAPTER 2

# Amy

A TYPICAL DAY IN MY OFFICE IS NEVER ROUTINE. The demand of seeing twenty-five to thirty-five patients between the hours of eight-thirty to five o'clock is physically and mentally exhausting for the entire staff: doctor, nurses, and receptionist. Pre-appointment responsibilities begin before patients arrive and include equipment and instruments preparation, setting up charts, checking overnight telephone messages, and reviewing lab, x-ray, and pathology reports. The whirlwind of talking to patients, doing exams, and dictating reports coincides with the incessant telephone calls—patients making appointments, checking on test results, asking about insurance claims or disability forms, as well as the calls from pharmacies, hospitals, and the ever-present drug representatives who are attempting to convince myself and my staff about the advantages of their therapeutic wares. The workload becomes more challenging and, at times, chaotic, as the day progresses. While the office staff readies the office, I am either performing surgery or making post-operative rounds.

This hectic and tense atmosphere is present on "good days" when there are no emergencies, unplanned procedures, and few unexpected visits from patients who need more time to discuss special crises, either medical or emotional in nature—the fifty-five-year-old with a positive breast biopsy for cancer, the single young adult career woman with acute genital herpes, the mother of three with an abnormal pap smear, or the seventy-three-year-old, vibrant and healthy, who has lost her husband of forty-eight years.

When I take a chart from the door rack, I quickly read and assess the purpose for the visit. Sometimes, but not always, I'm

9

able to use the nurse's notes as a guesstimate for the length of the appointment, although the words "annual exam" seldom indicate anything but a routine visit; but on one particularly demanding day, I knew the next patient would take more time than usual.

I mentally winced when I read, "five-year-old with vaginal pain." I stared at the chart before opening the door, took a deep breath, and entered the exam room knowing that a long and challenging visit was in store, not only for me, but for the mother and especially the new young gynecological patient. Even if the issue was not a serious one, diagnosing the problem would be easier than providing a non-traumatic "first" visit for this young girl. Be patient I told myself—and remember—quelling the child's fear is more important than my time.

Amy was the oldest daughter of one of my patients, a child I first met over a year ago when her mother, Veronica, was pregnant with her second baby. While I hadn't delivered Amy, she came to several of her mother's prenatal visits with a healthy curiosity. Her features were doll-like—rosy cheeks, blue eyes, and soft light brown hair. Usually, a doctor can assess the fabric of a family by observing the interaction between the child, her mother, and the occasional visits with the father. While parental love is the cornerstone of a child's security, self-esteem is fostered by the parent's mutual respect for each other as well as their attention to a child's emotional and intellectual development.

Amy was fortunate; Veronica and Bill were good parents with the right focus, intuition, and patience. Amy's congenial personality and appropriate social skills reflected a healthy family unit. But the situation was different now. Amy was no longer an innocent bystander, shielded from the intrusions of the hands, instruments, and needles of our office. She was now the patient in an environment different from her pediatrician's office. Absent were the colorful cartoon characters on the wallpaper, crayons to draw with in the waiting room, or the specialized nursing skills of a pediatric nurse—this was the medical world of her mother: adults with adult problems. No matter how well Veronica prepared Amy for the visit, or the familiar appearance of me, the doctor as the friendly person who takes care of her mommy, this office setting was unnatural and dealt with a part of her body that was socially "off-limits" to all but her family. When I entered the room, Amy's eyes didn't reveal anxiety as I expected, but expressed a natural suspicion with an underlying sense of curiosity for what was unknown.

"Hello, Veronica," I said as cheerfully as I could, while noticing her look of concern. "And hello, Amy," I said with a smile. "I remember when you used to come with your mommy when she was carrying your new sister."

Amy didn't smile, nor did she indicate any recollection of a happier time in my office, but she did look me straight in the eyes, a sign of a determined personality in spite of her young age.

"I understand you're having a little problem," I said euphemistically for her ailment, but her countenance remained unchanged. I swallowed hard and wondered if it would have been easier to find a hysterically sobbing child instead of one so resolute.

"Honey," Veronica said. "The doctor is speaking to you. Please tell him what you told me this morning."

No response. While adults reveal their emotions by body language and speech, Amy continued to stare at me without a verbal or physical response. As the doctor, I needed to become more assertive, but in a gentle way.

"Amy," I said slowly and calmly. "Your mommy told my nurse that you have something wrong with your vagina." Using correct anatomic terminology is the choice among today's parental generation—"privates," "down there," and cute euphemisms like "pee-pee" and "poo-poo" are not the words of enlightened parents. "Can you please tell me what you told the nurse and your mommy?" I asked in a hopefully non-threatening tone.

Amy lowered her head for a moment and slowly raised her eyes, revealing more fear than obstinacy. I was grateful when she said, "I don't want you to hurt me," with a whispered whimper.

"No, Amy," I said. "I don't want to hurt you. I want to help you. I'll explain everything that I need to do to find out what's bothering you. And your mommy will be with you the whole time."

With a sudden turn of her head, Amy looked at her mother for reassurance. Veronica, eyes moist, nodded approval. "The doctor wants to help you, dear. He's a nice doctor. Don't you remember when he let you hear Carrie's heartbeat when she was in my tummy, and he showed you pictures of Carrie with his special ultrasound machine?"

Now a faint smile came from Amy. "Uh huh," she said clearly. "That was fun."

"Yes," I said, hoping we were making progress, "and I never hurt your mommy or your baby sister, did I?"

"No," she whispered. "But I'm not in my mommy's tummy," she said with a pout.

How insightful and what a bright little girl she is, I thought. "You're right, Amy, but I can still help you and not hurt you, even though you are not in your mommy's stomach." Of course, I would have preferred to use the word "uterus," but the message needed to be explained clearly and without confusion. "Tell me what's bothering you first."

Most new patients are interviewed in my office before undressing for their examinations, but my nurses recognized the special situation and Amy sat straight up at the end of the exam table with a sheet folded neatly over her lap. She glanced towards the middle of the sheet and back at me.

"My vagina hurts. It started hurting while I was sleeping."

"I see." I was encouraged with the interaction and Amy's change of attitude, but I was still walking on thin ice and knew her defensives would return if she felt threatened. I weighed my words carefully before I spoke. "Is anything coming out of your vagina like water or paste?"

She hesitated for a moment and tilted her head to the side. "Yes. Like paste."

"Oh," I said nonchalantly, although I was given a huge piece of information. But how do I explain the nature of a pelvic exam to her? If I chose the wrong words, her resistance would return. I tried the direct approach—she was too smart for sugar-coating.

"Well, here's what we're going to do, Amy." I sat down on my stool and rolled closer to her. Now we were on an even eye level. "I'll examine your vagina, without hurting you, and find out why you have this paste coming out. Is that okay?"

She turned towards her mother again. Veronica nodded again. "Okay," she said quietly.

While Amy was cooperating, I needed to explain the nature of the exam clearly and without frightening her, and carry it out without causing discomfort. If I was unable to do so adequately and not discover the source of the vaginal pain and discharge, it would be necessary to admit Amy as an outpatient and perform an exam under anesthesia, a procedure I hoped to avoid.

With Veronica at the head of the table, and my nurse assisting me, I explained that I would be looking at her vagina with a special light and "touching her" without hurting her. Amy followed my instructions without any resistance. Her legs were too short for the stirrups, so we "frog-legged" her as she moved her bottom towards the edge of the table.

Slowly, I separated the labia and looked at the vaginal opening while telling Amy what I was about to do. The prepubescent vulva was inflamed with a white sticky discharge coming from the vaginal opening. Since the pre-puberty child has little estrogen production, the labia do not completely cover the vaginal opening with little protection against exposure to externally acquired bacteria and irritants. Added to this higher susceptibility is the neutral or alkaline acid-base status of a child's genitals. As the female enters puberty, anatomical development and a change in pH provide resistance to vaginal infections. The thinner and more delicate tissues of the pediatric female are especially prone to traumatic tears and irritation.

There was little doubt that Amy was symptomatic from a vulvo-vaginitis, or inflammation of the labia and vagina, but I needed to find out why. Pediatric vaginal infections can be caused by contamination from the gastrointestinal tract or skin, or, sadly, by sexually transmitted diseases. Knowing the family as well as I did, the latter was a low consideration. Amy remained cooperative as I continued to explain every step. I obtained cultures from the vaginal opening and a sample of the discharge to inspect microscopically. Since foreign bodies in the vagina are a common cause of pediatric vaginal infections, I needed to insert a small speculum to inspect the vaginal canal.

"Amy," I said slowly, "I need to put this tiny instrument into your vagina so I can find out why you have an infection." I held it up for her to see and asked if she wanted to hold it. Curiously, Amy took it and rubbed the shiny surface with her fingers.

"Looks like a toy," she said with a faint smile. The acceptance of the instrument as a non-threatening object was encouraging, but inserting it without causing pain was the real challenge. As I lubricated the instrument, a terrible thought entered my mind. Although I'd never seen a case, a condition called sarcoma botryoides, or an embryonal rhabdomyosarcoma, was a rare vaginal tumor, occurring during the first five years of life, arising from embryonic tissue that could extend to the uterus, lymph nodes, and eventually, malignant metastases. The cancer carried a poor prognosis even with surgery, radiation, and chemotherapy. The term "botryoides" comes from the Greek word "botrys" meaning "grapes" since the tumor resembles a polyp-like mass with the appearance of a bunch of grapes. I tried to rid this thought from my mind and concentrate on performing an exam while not creating pain or emotional trauma and, hopefully, make an appropriate diagnosis leading to a simple cure for this bright and beautiful little girl.

Amy was strong and brave and, as I inserted the small speculum, she flinched ever so slightly, and with calming words from her mother, I was able to insert the speculum past her hymen. Deliberately, I opened the speculum to visualize the world of a child's vaginal canal.

"Oh my," I said softly, hoping not to alarm Amy or her mother. I couldn't believe what I saw. "Looks like we found the problem," I said calmly. Emotionally, I was relieved, but intellectually, I was bewildered. Just inside the lower third of Amy's vaginal canal was not the dreaded "tumor of grapes" consistent with a rare pediatric cancer, but in fact a small green grape enveloped with inflammatory fluids from the reaction of the tissues to a foreign body. With great care, I took a pair of tweezers, grasped the displaced grape, and easily removed it.

"Well, well, well," I said with little creativity. "Look what I found," and held it up to show Amy and her mother.

Veronica gasped with surprise as well as embarrassment. Amy looked at the fruity culprit without any signs of emotion.

"I wonder how this got here, Amy," I said without criticism. It's not unusual for a young girl to place something in her vagina as a means of exploring her body and not as a sign of some strange, bizarre behavior. Usually, it's toilet paper, but the grape was unique. As relieved as I was to discover this, I was not prepared for Amy's response to my question.

"Oh," she said without any hesitation. "I know what happened with that grape."

"You do?" I asked incredulously.

Without any embarrassment or equivocation, Amy gave a cogent explanation.

"I was taking a bath and the grape fell from the ceiling into my vagina."

Mother and doctor glanced at each other smiling and without verbalizing any argument to Amy's explanation. What she did was natural, and what she said was simple child-like creativity and innocence.

A simple cream, medicated baths, and reassurance was all that was required to treat the infection. A few days later, when I followed up with Veronica by phone, Amy's pain and discharge had resolved without further complications.

The incident with Amy remained in the recesses of my mind until about seventeen years later when I took a chart from the rack and discovered it was the chart of Amy, now twenty-three years old and a senior in college. When I entered the room, I found a young adult with the beauty of the five-year-old who I first met. Amy matured into a sophisticated and dazzling looking young lady. She had not undergone a gynecological exam since the one I performed when she was five years old. Amy had a steady boyfriend and was responsible enough to return for an exam and discussion about birth control. Her visit was uneventful and she was gracious and appreciative. When I turned to leave the room, I hesitated for an instance, wondering if she would bring up the unusual incident from seventeen years ago. She didn't and I remained respectful, although I sensed there was a silent recognition of her previous visit to the office.

While there have been many "interesting" experiences in my medical career, Amy's situation remains a distinct and vivid one; and every now and then, when I pick up a grape, I look up at the ceiling—and smile.

# Chapter 3

# Jessica

FOR MOST DOCTORS, post-medical training is the most demanding time of his or her educational career. While the hours are modified for today's interns and residents, the training I obtained from 1976 to 1980 consisted of an eighty- to ninety-hour work week—years of sleep deprivation with unlimited physical and mental demands. During my internship, I made a little more than seven thousand dollars a year, a stipend well below the minimum wage; but as an obstetrics and gynecology resident, I gave up a normal life for four years of unparalleled training and hands-on clinical experience, providing the foundation for my medical expertise. While my fellow residents and I complained incessantly about the overwhelming work, silently we knew that at the completion of our training, we could handle any obstetrical or gynecological surgery, disease, or emergency—a feeling of confidence worth the years of sacrifice.

Two county hospitals existed in Houston during those years—the old Jefferson Davis Hospital, housing the city's obstetrical unit, pulmonary service, and rehabilitation medicine, and Ben Taub General Hospital, where all the other services were provided including the gynecology service. A night on call at either hospital was a choice of "pick your poison"—both places demanded a thirty-six hour stint of clinics, surgeries, and emergencies, fueled by a continuous consumption of mud-like coffee to maintain a therapeutic level of caffienated blood. While "Jeff Davis" recorded close to thirteen thousand births per year, the "Tub," our affectionate name for Ben Taub, was filled with gynecological emergencies requiring endless hospital admissions for gonorrheal pelvic inflammatory disease, messy miscarriages, ruptured tubal pregnancies, and the constant "gyne" consultations requested by the other medical services.

For me, the most emotionally uncomfortable demands were the rape cases. As an intern, my responsibilities were with adult rapes, requiring an examination to obtain legal evidence for the patient, as well as treating the physical trauma, providing preventive measures for pregnancy, and screening for sexually transmitted diseases. However, as a resident, I dealt with a more repulsive act of violence: the egregious trauma of pediatric rape. One night, I attended seven child molestations between the hours of 10 PM and 6 AM; and sadly, these innocent victims were the survivors, or at least children with a guardian or authority responsible enough to bring the child in for medical care. I shudder to think how many girls went unattended, or worse, were raped by family members who threatened them to remain silent. I did what I could for proper medical care, but the social services were few and emotional support for this "murder of the soul," unfortunately, was limited.

It was during my third year of training, confident with my obstetrical and gynecological skills, when I faced a particular horrifying case of pediatric sexual abuse. It was Christmas Eve, although nothing was festive at the hospital. Old and torn holiday ornaments, scattered throughout the wards, brought little cheer to the environment. All services were in high gear with infirmed patients: the poorly controlled diabetics with their vascular and kidney complications; the lonely burn patients in their isolated and dreary unit; the infected drug addicts sick but happy to have a bed and food; and the multitude of dying cancer patients sedated with IV medications. Not surprising, the emergency room remained a hot bed of activity, typical for a holiday. Like Friday and Saturday nights, holidays increased the usual madness— gun-shot wounds, stabbings, auto accidents, drug overdoses, and of course, the continuous rape cases. By the end of a usual night, the emergency room looked like a combat zone, splattered blood, needles, bandages, IVs, and stretchers everywhere, the aftermath of a medical hurricane blowing in medical debris.

It was already a tough night—I was closing an abdominal incision on an eighteen-year-old who almost died hemorrhaging from a ruptured tubal pregnancy.

"The ER keeps calling," the OR circulating nurse informed me matter-of-factly.

"Better get your butt down there when you're done," the chief resident told me. "And don't call me unless it's something really bad," he barked.

Great, I thought. It was only a little past eleven PM. The night was young. I finished the surgery, dictated the operative report, wrote orders, and checked on the patient in the recovery room. After four units of blood, she still appeared ghostly white. I went to the waiting room, surprised to find any family members present, and informed them of her condition. I learned quickly in my training not to take the elevators, since most were slow or not working at all. The stairs were the easiest way to negotiate the five floors, but the odor of urine and vomit, along with splashes of spit and blood on the walls, was the price you paid. By this time in my career, my senses were immune to the disgusting conditions. Once on the first floor, I walked through dirty corridors, entered the ER, now lined with sitting patients waiting for care, past the trauma rooms busy with gunshot wounds and auto accidents, to the GYN room located across the hall from a room reserved for the wheezing asthmatic as well as overdosed patients having their stomachs pumped, a most incongruous pairing.

The designated gynecological exam room was exclusive to our service, a place where we performed exams as well as the many D and C's for first trimester miscarriages, sometimes as many as ten per night. Since hospital staffing was inadequate, residents were doctor, anesthesiologist, nurse, lab, ward clerk, and orderly. When you got the routine down, you could do the whole thing in less than thirty minutes. Our motto was "learn one, do one, and teach one."

As I entered the room, I thought I was prepared to deal with the mechanics for a pediatric rape. My focus was on getting this "chore" done and moving on to another surgical case, this time a twenty-two-year-old with right lower quadrant pain, fever, and elevated white blood cell count, the bane of the gynecology resident. Many of these women had acute appendicitis instead of pelvic inflammatory disease, but the general surgery service was usually overwhelmed with trauma cases and any young female with this clinical presentation became our property. I needed to tend to this pediatric patient efficiently, fill out the necessary legal paperwork required by the police, and move on to this next case, but I was caught off guard when I entered the room.

Sitting on the exam table was a blond, fair skinned, blue eyed girl, around seven years of age, with her well groomed and dressed grandmother as the accompanying adult, an unusual scene. I introduced myself and found out the particulars. The young girl was staying at her grandmother's house for a few days during the winter school recess. Her grandmother didn't drive, but lived a short distance from the medical center and walked her granddaughter to the ER after the heinous incident.

The girl's name was Jessica, and surprisingly, an excellent historian, poised and collected for a child allegedly raped a few hours before. The details were horrifying—Jessica was pulled from her grandmother's porch by an unknown man, taken into his van, and sexually abused. Unlike any other pediatric victim, Jessica gave me the vile details without signs of fear or hysteria. Her grandmother, obviously shaken by the event, remained composed and supportive. After a brief exam looking for bites, bruises, and other signs of trauma, I explained to Jessica and her grandmother the need for a pelvic exam.

"That's where it hurts," she said softly, pointing towards her genitals. Yet, I wasn't prepared for the physical findings. With intercourse brutally forced upon her, Jessica sustained a tear in her vagina extending into the rectum.

My God, I thought. How could this child remain emotionally stable after such abuse? I swallowed hard and told myself to detach and remain professional. Jessica's injury would require surgery. With forced composure, I explained the details of the operation and, after receiving her grandmother's consent, wheeled Jessica to the OR, and repaired the extensive laceration. Her vaginal tissue was thin due to the lack of estrogen and required slow and meticulous suturing, particularly to the rectum. I hoped she would heal well without functional compromise to the vaginal canal or rectum, but Jessica's mental scarring was more of a concern to me.

I was not surprised to find Jessica's parents, as well as her grandmother, in the waiting room. As expected, her parents were deeply concerned for their daughter, but demonstrated composure as well as sincere appreciation for her care. What I had observed in the ER was what I saw postoperative, a little girl with bravery and maturity far beyond her chronological age. Jessica's postoperative recovery was uneventful and she went home with a follow-up appointment to the clinic.

A few weeks later, one of my fellow residents informed me that he tended to Jessica's postoperative visit and found the surgical repair healing well, free of infection or breakdown of the tissue. Fortunately, Jessica tested negative for any sexually transmitted diseases and was seeing a counselor. Though relieved to hear this, I knew that this special girl faced a long road of psychological recovery. However, I didn't expect to be involved with Jessica in an entirely different way.

Six months later, while in the clinic, I received a phone call from the county's district attorney's office. A man had been caught and arrested during another pediatric rape, and was suspected to be Jessica's offender. Now on trial, the assistant D.A. needed me in court that very afternoon to verify the medical findings. Apparently, she read the name in Jessica's chart incorrectly and subpoenaed the wrong resident for testimony. The D.A. asked the judge for a short recess and tracked me down. Although I needed to do my duty, I told her it would be impossible to leave the clinic on such short notice. Five minutes later, the clinic nurse informed me that the judge was on the phone. When I answered, he threatened me with contempt of court if I was not in the witness box within the hour. I shook my head in disbelief, found another resident to assume my duties, and headed for the courthouse.

The D.A., unapologetic for her error, quickly called the judge and the trial resumed. I saw Jessica, her parents, and grandmother, sitting calmly at the prosecution's table. The D.A. asked me to describe Jessica's findings, which I did as well as I could, followed by minimal questioning from the defense attorney. A few days later, I read the newspaper article describing the trial, Jessica's credible identification of her attacker, and the jury's guilty verdict followed by a long prison sentence. I have no doubt Jessica was a convincing and impressive witness.

Twelve years later, I introduced myself to a new patient, age nineteen, who was in for her first exam. Although usually good with names, it wasn't until I was well into the interview that I realized this Jessica was the one I had tended to during my residency. Her parents remembered my name, and recommended she see me for her first gynecological exam, although my practice was in another part of the city. While the details of her abuse were fuzzy, she recalled the hospitalization and the follow-up visits with a psychologist. Amazingly, when I examined her, there was no trace of residual trauma to her pelvis. Jessica was well adjusted, determined, and responsible. The professional counseling she received, as well as her loving family support, aided in her recovery from the vile victimization.

Jessica's story is consistent with a psychological observation that is sometimes difficult to explain. While many adults never recover well from what appears to have been a minor traumatic event, others show minimal psychological scarring from an incident seemingly catastrophic. For Jessica, her innate resiliency and family support provided the cornerstone for recovery. Sadly, most victims of unconscionable acts of violence carry the weight of mental trauma forever.

# PART III

# The Adolescent Years

# CHAPTER 4

# Cindy

MANY OF TODAY'S ADOLESCENTS are involved with extra-curricular activities, either through their schools, clubs, or religious groups. While keeping the teen busy is a healthy approach to their overall education and social development, too much activity can be detrimental to other concerns, such as schoolwork and family interactions. Added to this dilemma are the pressures many parents place on their children, a result when the child is viewed as an extension of a parent's identity. To "let go" and "be there" for their child, to love and support while not controlling, is a difficult concept to grasp for even the most enlightened parents. Nurturing is a strong instinct, and balancing it realistically is a formidable task. A teenager's mercurial moods, as well as their genetic and psychosocial influences, create a difficult parent/child conundrum.

Barbara, a patient of mine for many years, brought her sixteen-year-old daughter into the office to evaluate her sudden lack of menstrual periods. Cindy appeared healthy, had a pleasant affect, and was free of medical problems. She did well in school, had many friends, and was active in swimming and soccer. At five feet seven inches, Cindy was long and lean with a body mass index in the lower but normal range for her age. Cindy was not concerned about her periods, but Barbara, who was extremely overweight, appeared anxious.

"Cindy has always had normal periods, starting when she was thirteen," Barbara said while pointing a finger at me. "I never missed a period until I had my hysterectomy a few years ago. Maybe it's her thyroid?"

Barbara's life was stressful, mainly created by her own design. While I treated her with respect and professionalism, it was easy to discern her emotionally immature personality. Barbara was a frequent-flyer in my office, with complaints of pain, recurrent bladder and vaginal infections, and many other bodily ailments. Although she had demanding responsibilities as a hospital administrator, Barbara demonstrated many neurotic traits and continued to gain weight at an alarming rate. Divorced for six years, she desperately tried to balance her career while parenting her two children. Knowing the family on a social level provided me with helpful insights. Barbara, vindictive towards her ex-husband, did not hide her negative feelings from her children, creating more confusion for them in an environment already overwhelming. Cindy's father, Jim, missed being involved with his children on a daily basis. His caring and sensitive nature made him vulnerable to Barbara's selfish manipulations and spiteful wrath.

"Cindy," I asked. "Do you think you've lost weight over the past year?"

"Not much," she answered indifferently.

"Yes, she has," Barbara shouted. "She eats very little and works out for two hours every day even when soccer and swim seasons are over!"

Cindy rolled her eyes. "Mom, I eat okay!"

Not wanting a quarrel to develop between mother and daughter, I intervened.

"Cindy, are you feeling more stressed lately?"

She sighed and look me straight in the eyes. "No, not really. Well, you know, sometimes school and my sports wear me down, but no, I like what I'm doing."

"Hmmff," Barbara said loudly, "she's moody and won't listen to my advice."

Cindy's face turned red. "Mom!"

This was going nowhere. I needed to separate mother and daughter.

"That's okay, Cindy." I stood. "Let's do an exam and run some tests just to make sure there's no significant problem."

Cindy was cooperative and compliant. She was not sexually active and her exam was unremarkable. There was no clinical evidence to support a significant hormonal imbalance. I prescribed an oral progesterone tablet for ten days. Cindy responded with a small amount of spotting, confirming no structural female organ problems. I told Barbara and Cindy that while there was nothing seriously wrong, further weight loss could lower her estrogen level, possibly causing premature osteoporosis. Barbara accepted this reassurance and Cindy understood the need for proper nutritional intake particularly during times of increased exercise.

Occasionally, when I would see Barbara in the hospital corridors, she never mentioned any further problems with Cindy; but a few months later, Barbara brought Cindy in because of more weight loss. This time, Cindy did not look good. She was gaunt, pale, and had lost any spark in her usually bubbly personality. Her body mass index dropped below the lower levels consistent with her height and weight. Now I knew we had a serious problem. A bone mineral density test confirmed a reduction in bone mass. It was clear that Cindy was suffering from a form of anorexia called "Female Athlete Triad." This syndrome includes disordered eating habits, lack of periods, and bone loss due to a very low estrogen blood level associated with vigorous athletic training. While unlikely, some patients could progress to fractures, malnutrition, severe depression, and sadly, death. Most recover uneventfully but almost one-quarter of women with "Female Athlete Triad" will live with a chronic eating disorder associated with serious consequences.

Cindy needed help, but treatment wasn't that simple. Many of these patients come from family tendencies that include perfectionism, low self-esteem, and the need to control. While I considered prescribing estrogen to combat the bone loss, I elected to use a non-medication approach, including vitamin and calcium supplementation, nutritional counseling from a dietician, limitation of her exercise routine, and most importantly, both individual and family psychotherapy. At first, Barbara was reluctant to meet with Jim, but I urged her to do so for Cindy's health. Fortunately, the love for her daughter transcended her emotional obstacles and she agreed to the joint therapy sessions. I gave Barbara names of therapists whom I trusted and hoped for the best.

Cindy met twice a week with a psychologist with excellent psychotherapy skills. Once every other week, Barbara, Jim, and Cindy met together. Although the meetings were strained between parents, Cindy made progress, and fourteen months later, was back to her normal weight and monthly periods. She remained competitive in her sports and received a swimming scholarship to a state university.

Although Cindy did well, her mother did not. The mother/daughter relationship remained guarded, even though Cindy tried to reconcile their differences. Barbara became more depressed and, unfortunately, more obese, especially after Cindy's brother Seth decided to live with his dad during his sophomore year in high school. Jim got a chance to be the kind of father he was capable of being. He and Seth became great buddies, sharing golf, fishing, and their love for baseball. On a social level, I noticed a renewed Jim, content to parent his son.

Barbara stopped her therapy sessions soon after Seth moved out and became more bitter and neurotic than ever before. After much urging, I convinced Barbara to try an antidepressant, allowing her to become more functional, but it seemed tragic for an intelligent woman to lose so much in her life due to a need to control the people she loved and who loved her, while wallowing in self-pity. Who knows how Barbara's life would have turned out if she received the proper counseling when she was younger? Everyone has the opportunity to change their lives for the better, but it requires self-recognition, focus, and work.

Cindy was fortunate to climb out of her destructive behavior. Eating disorders among teenage girls can become a dangerous medical and psychological challenge that can only be overcome with a strong inner fortitude and the right professional help. Cindy's recovery was a credit to her determination as well to sound psychotherapy.

# CHAPTER 5

# Carrie

FOR FEMALE ADOLESCENTS, primary and preventive health care requires an understanding of behavioral habits as well as traditional medical attention. For some teenage girls, the transition from childhood to adulthood is relatively calm and uneventful, but for others, the development of psychological, physical, and cognitive maturity may be a difficult journey. It is estimated that seventy-five percent of adolescent and young adult deaths stem from causes that are preventable. While the bulk of guidance comes from the home, a health care provider can participate in a young woman's passage from childhood to adulthood.

Part of an adolescent's involvement in risky behaviors, such as poor nutritional habits, smoking, alcohol and drug use, driving while intoxicated, and early sexual activity, occurs because there is an assumption of invulnerability. Most teenagers believe they are different from others and not liable to the risks that threaten their peers. Physical developments are usually not in phase with psychological and cognitive maturity. Eventually, discretion develops when intellectual and emotional resources permit the adolescent to perceive reckless behavior as dangerous. I witness many adolescents who subject themselves to risky activity, while the mother, usually one of my patients, looks on with frustration and anxiety.

Many mothers ask when they should "bring their daughters in" for a gynecological exam. The old adage "not until she is having problems" does not comply with the newer proactive and preventive approach in female adolescent health. Between the ages of thirteen and fifteen, a young woman should visit an ob-

stetrician-gynecologist, and then annually. The first visit is a cru-
cial one—a visit without an exam (unless medically indicated) to
discuss normal adolescent development, screening for physical,
emotional, and behavioral conditions, and assessment of proper
immunizations, as well as health promotion and risk reduction
strategies with the patient as well as the parent(s).

Although every daughter/parent relationship is unique, developing a foundation for confidentiality is the most important issue during this visit. It must be firmly stated and adhered to by the
office staff, patient, and the parent(s) in order for the adolescent to
feel a trust with the physician. While the teenager is encouraged
to involve her parent(s) with health and health care decisions, the
proverbial door must be left open for the adolescent to confide
privately with the health professional and accept medical advice.
While state and local statutes regarding rights of minors to health
care services differ, federal law insures confidentiality for the patient. The federal Health Insurance Portability and Accountability
Act (HIPAA) went into effect on April 14, 2003 to insure that the
use and disclosure of medical information remains confidential.
Physician and office staff are required to maintain this confidentiality and ensure that professional services are not compromised
by either legal and/or economic constraints.

After twenty years of private practice, I began seeing a different kind of "new" patient—a female who I once helped birth
into this world. Knowing that the doctor was their mother's
obstetrician mitigates some of the anxiety associated with a first
gynecological exam. While it is an honor to provide care for these
young women, it never fails to stir a bittersweet moment—the
transition from infant to a young and vibrant adult, and the sad
reality check of my own age. This was poignantly displayed when
a hospital administrator greeted me in the hallway one day and
related a humorous, but interesting, story to me.

"I know you don't remember," she said, "but you delivered
my daughter eighteen years ago today!"

After the usual remarks about "time flies!" and "isn't it amaz-
ing how fast they grow up!," the administrator related the comment her daughter had made at breakfast that morning. After

the "gushy" statements about how beautiful she had become and how difficult it was to believe that she was born eighteen years ago, the daughter innocently replied, "Gee, Mom. Do you think the doctor who delivered me is still alive today?" For the rest of the day, I felt the way I did when I received my first AARP offer in the mail. But not all cases are light or happy.

Susan, an established patient, brought her fourteen-year-old in for her first visit. Carrie was a pleasant young teenager, a little shy, but sociable, and she, Susan, and I discussed several issues: exercise, good study habits, proper nutrition, forming healthy relationships with peers, hazards of alcohol and drugs, and encouragement for abstinence as the best protection from sexually transmitted diseases and pregnancy. While I encourage all teens to discuss medical or social problems with their parents, I emphasized to both the need to maintain confidentiality regarding Carrie's medical care within my office. They agreed. Carrie was healthy and other than minor acne and her dislike for orthodontic braces, she had no apparent medical, psychological, or social problems.

The next year, Carrie came with her mother again; this time the fifteen-year-old was taller, without braces, and a bit "sassy" with her remarks. She never made eye contact with me when I asked questions, but instead, gave short responses reflecting an annoyed attitude. Susan appeared anxious and commented at the end of the visit, "You know, Carrie really didn't want to come in today."

This was a predictable moment—a young teenager rebelling from confusion about her identity and from the pressures that overwhelm an adolescent whose psychological and intellectual reserves are not well developed yet. Much to the surprise of both mother and daughter, I asked politely for Susan to leave so Carrie and I could have a private conversation. Susan appeared uneasy.

"Well, I'm not sure why I need to," she said, eyes darting from Carrie to me.

I tried to find the right balance of compassion and professionalism. I leaned forward. "Remember the important agreement we made during last year's first visit? Carrie's medical care is confidential." Now Carrie was staring at me with wide eyes.

"Carrie, is it all right with you if your mother leaves and you and I chat for a little while?"

Carrie swallowed, looked at her mom, and said "Sure, I really don't care." While her façade revealed indifference, I suspected she was really scared and unsure.

Reluctantly, Susan left and Carrie sat in silence while staring at her shoes.

"Carrie, I just want to reassure you that you can tell me anything that concerns you without anyone else knowing what we discuss in this office. I told you that last year and I'm telling you this again. And that goes even after you leave this office." I leaned back in my chair. "I encourage you to discuss problems with your parents, but if it is too uncomfortable for you, please have one of your parents, or a friend, bring you to the office and we'll discuss it in confidence. And that goes for my staff also. They cannot give information out to anyone without your permission."

Carrie looked at me for an instance and lowered her head. "Okay. But I have nothing to tell you."

"That's perfectly all right," I said hoping to reassure her. "But if you ever do need to talk to me about something personal, you have that right without anyone else having knowledge of what we discussed."

Carried nervously rubbed her hands without responding. Obviously, she was uncomfortable and wanted to leave. But I needed to add a caveat.

"Carrie, the only thing that would break our confidentiality is if I believed there might be any risk of harm to you or to others. That's a moral principle I must stick to."

Carrie stared at her hands for a few moments before looking at me. "Can I leave now?"

I smiled. "Yes, Carrie. You may. Call me if you need me. If not, I'll see you next year.

After she left, I wondered if Carrie and Susan understood the importance of patient confidentiality; but it wasn't until a few months later, when Susan came for her annual exam, that I received my answer. At the conclusion of the exam, Susan confided in me: "I just want you to know that I appreciate your meeting with Carrie. At first, I couldn't understand why you excluded me, but after discussing it with my husband, we agreed that this is the way it ought to be." She sighed. "While we hope Carrie will be able to discuss anything with us, we also feel comfortable knowing that she can come to you if she chooses."

I thanked Susan for her understanding.

"By the way, how is Carrie?"

Susan raised her eyebrows. "I'm not quite sure. Some days she seems fine—happy, eating well, exercising, studying hard." She frowned. " But, sometimes she's extremely moody, eats nothing but junk food, and argues with me, my husband, and her younger brother."

Typical adolescence or something else?, I thought.

"Do you think she needs to see me?"

Susan shook her head. "Not sure. When I try to talk with her, she says little and gets annoyed when I ask about her friends or school."

I nodded. There was little I or Susan could do at this point.

"Well, call me if you have any concerns, Susan," I said hoping it sounded reassuring.

I didn't hear from either Carrie or Susan for the next several months. While there are several appointment "no shows" and reschedules per day, I noticed a cancellation next to Carrie's name for her next annual visit. At first, it didn't seem significant since a teenager's busy schedule can create conflicts, but I became concerned when Carrie missed her third appointment, this time without a call to cancel. A few weeks later, my apprehensions were validated when Susan called the office to talk to me about a "problem" with Carrie.

"She's been acting strange for the past few months." Susan looked tired and her eyes were puffy. "Carrie won't listen to us, stays out well past her curfew on the weekends, speaks to her boyfriend for two or three hours every night on the phone, has lost weight, and looks unhealthy. Even her grades are down." She shook her head. "We've tried everything, but she won't communicate with me or my husband."

I listened but had little to suggest. Either Carrie's behavior stemmed from adolescent rebellion or from something more serious. Time would tell, but I asked Susan to continue to urge Carrie to see me. It wasn't until a few months later that I discovered the reasons for Carrie's actions when I noticed her name penciled in on the patients schedule.

"Did Susan call to make an appointment for Carrie?" I asked my receptionist.

"Uh, uh. It was Carrie who called."

I raised my eyebrows. "Did she say what for?"

"No, she wouldn't tell me. Just said it was an emergency." She looked at me. "She was crying."

I rubbed my chin. What was going on?

While Carrie was reticent during her last visit, this time, she was communicative. Carrie cried and spoke with a new openness, although the issues I heard were not good ones. One of Carrie's friends, an older girl who dropped out of school, had overdosed the night before. Although her friend was resuscitated, she was in serious condition and on a respirator in the hospital's ICU. Although I didn't know her friend personally, I recognized her name as the daughter of a couple I knew socially. As a doctor, I felt empathy for Carrie's friend and her parents; as a father, I was horror-stricken.

Carrie was scared. When asked specifics, she admitted to alcohol and drug use, as well as sexual promiscuity without contraception. She agreed to an exam and tolerated it well after I explained the details. She was not pregnant, but anemic from her poor dietary habits. A few days later, her cervical culture tested positive for chlamydia, a sexually transmitted infection. Carrie was treated and counseled appropriately. I urged her to talk with her parents who loved her and would support her through these difficult times. While I asked Carrie to practice abstinence, I did discuss contraception with her. I hoped she would change her ways.

Carrie did change, although it was someone else's tragedy that led to Carrie's enlightenment. Sadly, her friend didn't recover from the overdose. A few days later, I attended the funeral along with many other parents, children, and friends. As I scanned the room of people in the chapel, I studied their faces. Did they share the same worry I did—and what about the kids—were they sad, angry, or just confused? I wondered how this young woman's death would affect all who knew her. Everyone present would process this in their own way and time.

Carrie turned her life around. She became a good student again, took better care of herself physically, and, while conflicts with her parents continued, she eventually told them about her risky experiences. Fortunately, Susan and her husband remained supportive in spite of their disappointments and Carrie found it easier to talk with them and ask for advice.

Carrie is a young adult now with a responsible career and in a healthy relationship. Her adolescence, like most teenagers, was stormy, but parents must never give up and continue to love their children unconditionally. Perhaps the author James Baldwin stated it best when he wrote, "Children have never been good at listening to their elders, but they have never failed to imitate them."

## PART IV

# Young Adults

## CHAPTER 6

# Janet and Lisa

As tumultuous as the adolescent years are, a young adult female has her own set of conflicts and challenges. While armed with a limited level of maturity, this individual must learn to balance a world of autonomy with the struggles of new life experiences and more demanding responsibilities. Most young adult women "find" themselves in their early to late twenties, but not without facing difficult decisions about issues that may have significant influences on their lives.

When a doctor practices obstetrics long enough, he or she may have the opportunity to take care of those they delivered. While I made the decision to stop obstetrics after the first ten years of practice, it remains satisfying to meet these baby girls as teens or young adults. Such was the case of fraternal twins, born during my first year of practice.

Janet and Lisa were delightful people—attractive, intelligent, and energetic. Their parents, Bob and Michelle, provided a loving environment for them, while passing on their clever wit and optimistic attitudes as well. When the twins were sixteen, an amusing scene occurred one Friday night when my wife and I were dining at a local restaurant. While savoring our meal, Janet and Lisa approached our table and asked politely if I was the doctor they thought I was. Although I didn't know who these girls were, I acknowledged I was that person. After introducing themselves, Janet said, "You delivered us sixteen years ago," followed by Lisa who said, "And our parents want their money back!" As we all laughed, many patrons turned and stared, either amused or annoyed by our levity.

It wasn't until the twins were twenty-three years old when I saw them again—this time for routine gynecological exams. Both had graduated from college and were entering different careers, and were counseled about contraceptive options and their benefits and risks. Janet preferred to use condoms, while Lisa chose an oral contraceptive. Both appeared to be healthy and had normal exams and Pap smears. Neither Janet nor Lisa was involved in any destructive behaviors, such as alcohol or drug abuse, and both seemed discreet when choosing partners. I wished them luck with their new careers and expected to see them in one year.

About six months later, Janet came for a visit with her sister, but it was not routine. Both seemed anxious and it didn't take long to confirm their fears.

"What seems to be the problem, Janet," I asked while noticing apprehension in her eyes.

Her words were barely audible. "Doctor, I'm late on my period."

Today, most patients have access to a home pregnancy test, but this wasn't available at that time. Women's intuition is powerful, especially when suspecting pregnancy. I sighed before pursuing further questioning.

"Janet, have you been using contraception?"

She lowered her head. "Yes, condoms, but ... but we may have forgotten one time."

I nodded. "Any breast tenderness, nausea, or tiredness?"

"Yes," she whispered. "All of those."

"I see," was my obligatory professional response, despite my heartfelt concern for her and her devoted sister sitting motionless in a chair. My nurse came into the exam room and showed me the positive pregnancy test.

"Okay, Janet," I said as calmly as possible. "Your test is positive."

She was approximately six weeks pregnant. As a physician, I need to maintain professional demeanor, and while my personal feelings and judgments are factors from which I cannot detach, they must not play a role in my clinical decision-making or in the way I choose my words when communicating to my patients.

Janet had made a decision that if pregnancy were confirmed, she would choose to terminate it because of her young age, new career, and the "casual" relationship with her new boyfriend. While Lisa was supportive to her sister, intuitively I believed she would have chosen to have the baby. I asked Janet to think it over for a few more days, and discuss it either with her parents, a religious leader, counselor, or all three, before making her final decision.

The abortion issue in this country is marked by significant moral pluralism that will continue to create fervent debates between those in favor of a woman's right to choose and those against the termination of an unborn life. As a physician, I respect the need for those in my profession who perform abortions under medically and psychologically safe methods and conditions, as well as the patient's choice concerning what is best for her. While I was taught how to perform abortions in my residency, I chose not to in private practice—partly because of the moral quandary and partly because of an event that happened when I first began practice. When I saw cardiac movement in my first unborn son under ultrasonic imaging, I knew that abortions would not be part of my services. Yet, I feel strongly that my patients deserve appropriate counseling and referrals to doctors or clinics providing pregnancy terminations.

Janet's dilemma bothered me from a professional perspective as well. Had I not advised her adequately or given her enough time to discuss options at her initial visit? I knew that elective pregnancy terminations reflected a breakdown in our social environment and educational system. Improvement in reproductive guidance, as well as accountability for both contraceptive and sexually transmitted disease protection, was a societal responsibility. Young adults need to take on adult responsibilities; but when a woman has an unplanned pregnancy, as in Janet's case, her health care provider must give options without introducing personal bias.

A few days later, Janet called and told me her decision. Fortunately, she spoke with her parents and met with a pregnancy counselor. While I knew Janet would experience a rocky emotional road after a termination, I was pleased she sought parental and professional advice and was acceptable to psychological support. Janet would experience transient, self-limited feelings of guilt as well as loss, but would probably recover without significant mental scars. I referred her to a colleague who performed pregnancy terminations. When I saw her a few weeks later, she had recovered without any medical problems and elected to take a low-dose oral contraceptive.

A year later, the twins returned for their annual visits. Both were doing well and tolerating their oral contraceptives without problems. I am a firm believer in "the pill," not only as a contraceptive, but for the other non-contraceptive benefits: regulation of menstrual periods, decreased menstrual flow and menstrual cramps, reduction in both uterine and ovarian cancer, as well as protection from endometriosis, pelvic infections, and osteoporosis. For some of my patients, acne is significantly improved with today's pill. While some women don't tolerate the pill well, others enjoy its many benefits. One drawback to the pill is the need to be compliant when taking it, since missing a low-dose pill can result in "breakthrough bleeding," or the worse scenario, an unwanted pregnancy. Much to my amazement, that's what happened to Lisa just three months later.

Lisa came to the office with her sister, now facing the same problem Janet had less than two years before. My exam confirmed an eight-week pregnancy. Lisa admitted to forgetting several pills the previous month and not using backup contraception. While the sisters were different in their goals and personalities, this strange coincidence was disturbing.

This time Janet was the main supporter and her previous experience gave her more insight about an unplanned pregnancy. While Janet felt strongly about terminating her pregnancy, she knew her sister's decision had to be her own one. It felt strange to counsel Lisa as I had done with Janet, again questioning whether I was delinquent with my advice to the twins. Yet Lisa had been irresponsible with her contraception compliance and accepted the consequences. She agreed to discuss this with her parents and call me with her decision. I remember her phone call a few days later.

"Hello, Lisa," I said upbeat hoping it didn't sound too contrived.

"Hi, Doctor," she replied. But I could "read" her tone of voice. While patients' mannerisms, body language, and facial expressions can provide great insight into that person's emotional milieu, the voice can be just as revealing. Lisa sounded focused and determined.

"I want to have this baby and find a caring couple to adopt the child."

Although not what I expected, I knew Lisa had thought it through well.

"Okay Lisa. I respect your decision."

She paused before continuing.

"Doctor, I know what kind of people would make good parents."

I didn't expect to hear her next comment.

"I want the couple to be like my mom and dad ... parents who will care well for this child. You know, parents that will love him or her unconditionally. That'll make my choice an easier one to accept."

While I knew raising the twins was difficult at times, Lisa's validation for her parent's upbringing was refreshing to hear after a long day of patients' complaints and cynicism. Although I was surprised by the choice, her mature and reasonable logic seemed appropriate and sensible.

Janet made her decision to terminate her pregnancy based on her set of circumstances, yet Lisa had done the same and her choice didn't seem to be influenced by her sister's decision. As a physician, my role was to support her choice. Since I no longer performed deliveries at this time, I referred Lisa to an obstetrician for prenatal care and gave her a list of adoption agencies.

Based not only on curiosity, but also on my concern for Lisa's welfare, I kept close tabs on her pregnancy and outcome. Lisa had an uneventful delivery and chose the adopting couple after several interviews with prospective parents. Lisa returned to see me six weeks later, and decided on the contraceptive injection instead of the pill.

The twins returned a year later for their annual exam. Both were doing well socially and with their careers. Janet finished graduate school in business studies and was working for a small company with potential growth. She had a steady partner for the past six months and appeared relaxed and happy. Lisa was working for a company which recognized her creative energy. Like Janet, she had a steady partner. After their exams, the twins showed me photographs of the little girl Lisa brought into this world. The adopting parents sent pictures and letters on a regular basis and offered an open invitation for their visits any time. Janet considered herself, rightfully, to be the little girl's aunt and enjoyed the feedback as much as her sister. I had no doubt that Lisa and Janet, in some way, would be part of this little girl's life.

Hypothetically, if Janet had not terminated her pregnancy, but given her child up for adoption, would the circumstances be the same? Or, would her decision have been different some other time in her life? Or would the choice have remained the same? While it is difficult to speculate on such issues, one thing seemed certain to me—her choice was the right one at that time. What appeared to be an unwanted situation for Lisa was now a fortunate one for her, Janet, the adoptive parents, and especially, for the well-being of this child.

# CHAPTER 7

# Sarah

LIKE SEVERAL "SUN BELT" CITIES, many cold climate transplants call Houston home, delighted with the mild winters and plentiful sunny days—no more snow, slush, or prolonged cloudy skies.

Sarah came to my practice when she was twenty-seven years old. A native of Chicago, she easily adapted to the hectic, but friendly pace of the nation's fourth largest city. The low rent and housing made her new salary seem like a major raise from the stipend she received in Illinois. Sarah adapted quickly to her new environs, making many friends and optimistically looking towards the future. She was personable, smart, and lived a healthy lifestyle. On occasions, I would see her at my fitness center where she would tell me, excitingly, about her career advancements. Like many young adults, Sarah saw opportunities for success and a focus on living life well.

Since the office clinic days are arranged well in advance, an "add on" patient to an already saturated schedule can be disruptive. While some of these "emergencies" turn out to be minor medical issues, some can be serious.

When I took Sarah's folder from the door rack, I knew she had been added to the schedule. The night before a clinic day, I preview the next day's patient list, hoping to prepare for necessary procedures. Some days appear tame and manageable on paper but turn out to be physically and mentally exhausting, while others look like "killers," but instead, flow smoothly and remain on schedule. This particular morning was not going well—one post-op with an unexplained fever and many patients with a multitude of complaints. Added to this load was a hospital department meeting at noon.

The nurse's note on Sarah's chart read "severe abdominal pain" and nothing else. The definition of "severe" is arbitrary, and a person's perception of pain is dependent on many factors, including the individual's pain threshold, emotional fortitude, as well as social and cultural influences; but when I entered the room, one look at Sarah was enough—her pain was intense.

Sarah's legs were curled up to her chest, not a good sign, and her temperature was 102.6 degrees. While Sarah was in acute distress, I needed to ask her several questions. Slowly, I got the medical history—increasing abdominal pain over the past two days, associated nausea, vomiting, and fever. Her gynecological history was negative—normal menstrual periods on an oral contraceptive. A pregnancy test was negative and her urinalysis was clear of any infection.

"Sarah, have you noticed any vaginal discharge?"

"Yes," she whispered. "And it has a bad odor."

I needed to find out more. "When was the last time you had relations?"

She was slow to respond. "Four days ago."

"Did you use condoms?"

Her words were barely audible. "No."

"Was this a steady partner of yours?" I asked professionally and without judgment.

She paused and shook her head. "No, I met him Saturday night at a club." Even though she was in much pain, I still detected a tone of regret and embarrassment in her voice.

I put the pieces together quickly after the exam. Sarah's abdomen was extremely tender, particularly in the lower half. A pelvic exam revealed foul-smelling white discharge as well as an inflamed cervix. I obtained cultures for gonorrhea and chlamydia, both sexually transmitted bacteria. But most revealing was the pelvic exam. When I palpated her uterus and ovaries, Sarah responded with a disturbing scream while sliding up the exam table. I apologized for hurting her.

"Sarah," I said slowly, hoping not to stir further anxiety, "you have a pelvic infection. While we can try to treat you with antibiotics on an outpatient basis, I believe it would be better being admitted to the hospital and receiving intravenous antibiotic therapy as well as pain meds." I didn't mention the potential complications like a pelvic abscess requiring surgery, or the formation of adhesions, or scar tissue, leading to chronic pelvic pain or infertility.

Sarah swallowed. "Okay," she said quietly. "Whatever you think is best."

Upon admission, blood tests revealed an elevated white blood cell count. While I could not rule out an acute appendicitis or a ruptured ovarian cyst, my clinical interpretation was pelvic inflammatory disease (PID), a broad diagnosis indicating a sexually transmitted disease. A pelvic ultrasound revealed fluid in her pelvis, but no evidence of ovarian cysts. While I couldn't be certain her problem was PID, I stuck to my clinical diagnosis and began appropriate IV antibiotic treatment.

While PID is not common in my practice, I had years of experience diagnosing and treating this gynecological condition as a resident. The county hospital ward was always filled with young women with PID. In the 1970s, gonorrhea was the major bacterial insult, but today chlamydia is more common, and unfortunately, harder to detect and even more destructive to the fallopian tubes.

Several weeks during my second-year residency, I noted an unusual number of PID admissions. Even more startling was the number of attractive females from California who were ending up on our service. It didn't take long to find out why. A major motion picture was being filmed in Houston, and apparently, some young stud or studs were infecting the female "extras" with a virulent form of gonorrhea. These women did not have health insurance, hence their admission to the county hospital.

Fortunately, Sarah did respond quickly to the intravenous antibiotics. Her fever, abdominal pain, and vaginal discharge resolved over the next few days and her white blood cell count returned to normal. The cultures I obtained in the office came back positive for gonorrhea as well as chlamydia. Sarah was sent home with oral antibiotic treatment and pain medication. I counseled her about the nature of her disease and asked her to notify her partner.

When I saw her one week later, Sarah looked like her old self again. Other than a mild vaginal yeast, or fungal infection resulting from the antibiotics, the abdominal examination was normal. While Sarah still felt pain during the pelvic exam, the degree was dramatically reduced from her initial exam. Although she would always carry a mental scar from this trauma, I hoped the infection hadn't left her pelvis with other scars leading to regrettable consequences.

Several weeks later, Sarah returned for a follow-up visit. She had a normal period without cramps and no urological or gastrointestinal complaints. In spite of significant improvement, Sarah still had some residual pain when I examined her pelvis. An ultrasound revealed slight "swelling" to Sarah's fallopian tubes, but no tumors or cysts were found during imaging. Could this still be some inflammation remaining from her infection, I thought?

Repeat cultures were negative and Sarah adamantly denied having relations since the hospitalization. I sent her home with an anti-inflammant for pain relief and didn't see her again until six months later when she returned for a follow up exam. She was doing well at work and told me about a new boyfriend she met a month ago.

"You know, doctor, I'm afraid to have relations with this guy, even though I'm crazy about him."

"Sarah," I said, "just be patient. You had a serious infection coupled with a personal violation. When the time is right, good things will happen."

Sarah agreed and appreciated the support. About seven months later, she returned for her routine Pap smear. She looked cheerful and healthy, and excitedly, told me about her engagement. The wedding was scheduled for the following year. Sarah continued on her oral contraceptive and maintained normal periods except for one problem.

"Doctor," she said with a look of concern. "I have a question."

"What is it, Sarah?"

She tightened her lips. "Well, sometimes, when Lyle and I make love, I feel pain."

My concern was confirmed during the exam. Sarah remained tender when I palpated her tubes and ovaries.

"Sarah," I said as professionally as I could. "This may represent some damage from the pelvic infection." She was intuitive enough to have sensed this possibility. We agreed to observe her symptoms and to call if the condition worsened. Since her pain was not constant, a conservative approach was appropriate.

Sarah and Lyle were married, bought a house, and made a home with his dog and her cat. The next two annual visits were unremarkable except for Sarah's occasional pain during intercourse. Their careers continued to be successful and the couple's married life seemed happy and loving. But when Sarah returned again, it wasn't for a routine visit.

Sarah and Lyle were trying to conceive for the past nine months. While infertility testing is usually begun after a year of unprotected intercourse, my concern was magnified by her previous medical history. Sarah had bought a urine indicator kit confirming ovulation at the appropriate time in her cycle. Lyle agreed to a semen analysis which it was normal. Sarah needed an x-ray test called a hysterosalpingogram, or HSG, in order to assess the status of her fallopian tubes. As I feared, it confirmed that both tubes were blocked and filled with fluid, a condition called bilateral hydrosalpinx.

Since my practice has evolved into a sub-specialized one, consisting of menopausal medicine, female urinary incontinence, and pelvic surgery, I don't have the time or expertise to evaluate infertility patients past preliminary testing. Additionally, I find the emotional intensity involved with infertility conditions more demanding than other gynecologic problems. Fortunately, our medical center has an infertility specialist who is warm, compassionate, and excellent in her work. Sarah made an appointment to see Dr. Diane Roberts who recommended surgery to assess her fallopian tubes. Dr. Roberts and I discussed the possibilities: if the tubes were beyond repair secondary to severe damage, it would be best to surgically remove them to reduce Sarah's pain as well as increase the possibility of successful in-vitro fertilization. Sarah agreed.

On the morning of her surgery, I spoke with Sarah and Lyle in the preoperative room. She was naturally nervous, but emotionally prepared for the outcome.

"Do the best you can, Doctor." She smiled. "I trust your judgment."

I grasped her hand and gave her a reassuring nod.

The laparoscope doesn't lie. Sarah's tubes were beyond repair, dilated like tubular balloons from her previous infection. Dr. Roberts and I successfully removed her tubes via the scope and Sarah made an uneventful recovery. But now she faced a more difficult challenge—the time, expense, and emotionally draining efforts of in-vitro fertilization. Not only are perseverance and a bit of luck needed, but a couple's support for one another remains essential. After three attempts, Dr. Roberts made a successful implant from one of Sarah's fertilized "eggs" into her uterus. The couple was ecstatic and Sarah's pregnancy was uneventful. She delivered a healthy eight-pound two-ounce boy named Austin.

Over the next few years, Sarah would see me for routine visits. Her son was healthy and the joy of the couple's life. As happy as I was for this family, I knew many infertile couples who did not have success. While technology provides extraordinary advances, it still cannot change the vicissitudes of life—the unpredictable nature of events. Sarah was fortunate.

A few years later, Lyle received a promotion requiring a transfer to St. Louis. Before the relocation, Sarah came to give us her farewells. As a token for her appreciation, she gave me a framed photo of herself, Lyle, and their son that remains on a bookcase in my office. On some days, when the workload is exhausting and the patient problems overwhelming, I peek at the photo, smile, and continue my day with renewed strength and purpose.

# PART V

# The Pregnant Years

# CHAPTER 8

# Lucy

EARLIER IN MY PRACTICE, days consisted of a demanding office schedule followed by many nights of birthing babies. A good night's sleep was a rare event. While I recall interesting cases, most obstetricians learn that no pregnancy is ever just routine.

Lucy's prenatal care seemed straightforward. On her first visit, I found a healthy twenty-six year-old, pregnant for the first time. Her husband, Kevin, seemed affable and responsible. They asked relevant questions during that first visit, but as her pregnancy progressed, I began to realize how wrong I was about my initial impressions.

An obstetrician has the opportunity to see many facets of a person and their relationships. Husbands or partners come to the office for various reasons: concern, love, and support—the healthy ones. But others come because their significant other demands their time and attention, or sadly, because the male partner wants to control the situation. Domestic violence is a widespread problem affecting women of all ages, races, and socioeconomic levels, and is a major cause of physical injuries, emotional illness, and even homelessness among the female population. Eight to twelve percent of American women in an existing relationship experience at least one episode of domestic assault, nearly five million women per year are abused, and almost two million experience severe abuse.

There exists a vast array of violent acts—intimidations, throwing objects, pushing, kicking, beating, hitting, and threats to use a weapon as well as its use. Unfortunately, sexual assault remains a common egregious act. Nonviolent abuses include verbal attacks as well as deprivation of money, food, transportation, and even access to medical care leading to depression, fear, social isolation, and psychosomatic complaints. While every situation is unique, there appears to be a pattern among abusers. The "tension building phase" involves blaming, arguing, and jealousy which intensifies the anger. This may escalate to the "battering phase" with the use of verbal threats, physical violence, or sexual abuse. The last phase may be a reason a woman stays in an abusive relationship. The so-called "honeymoon phase" is the most psychologically difficult to comprehend for those not exposed to domestic violence. The abuser may deny the acts, make excuses for his behavior, blame the partner, alcohol, or drug addiction for his actions, or even apologize, buy gifts, and make promises never to cause harm again. Unfortunately, most abused women endure multiple episodes of violence before seeking medical, criminal, legal, or social assistance.

Our office keeps pamphlets entitled "Help for Women in Abusive Relationships" in the restrooms. In this booklet are quotes from women who have managed to escape and survive domestic violence. Examples include the following:

"He kept telling me I deserved to get hurt, and for a long time I believed him."

"I was more afraid of how he'd hurt me if I left than I was of what was happening at home."

"He kept saying he couldn't live without me! I thought, I can't leave him when it would make him feel so bad."

"I thought it [the abuse] was just because I couldn't do anything right. If I could just do better, he'd stop. But no matter how hard I tried, he didn't stop. The best thing I did was to get away."

"He kept begging me to forgive him, promising he'd never hurt me again. I guess I believed him, over and over, because I didn't want the children not to have a father if we left."

"If I left him, I didn't think I could make it on my own. Where would I go? How would I earn a living?"

All these statements reflect the confusion and fear an abused woman faces within a violent domestic relationship. It takes great strength and support to leave the abuser and be on one's own.

Although Lucy and Kevin appeared to be a functionally healthy couple, it didn't take long to find out otherwise.

At Lucy's next prenatal visit, Kevin attended as well. While we encourage husbands/partners to participate, it seemed odd that he came again, particularly since he had a high-pressured job at a car dealership. Lucy seemed reserved and Kevin asked most of the questions, all appropriate. Perhaps this was their relationship, I thought. Kevin was in control and Lucy preferred to remain quiet, maybe submissive. Nothing seemed unusual or odd. Retrospectively, I didn't see the red flags.

Kevin came to the next three visits. Lucy would either answer questions with a simple "yes," "no," or "I'm not sure," or Kevin would answer for her. Lucy was doing well physically, but the feelings weren't there—happiness, worry, confusion, and anger, all part of a normal pregnant woman's emotional milieu. Instead, Lucy seemed devoid of reactions, especially when we heard the baby's heartbeat on her second visit and when an ultrasound revealed fetal activity on a subsequent visit. Kevin not only spoke for Lucy, but felt for her as well. Perhaps, I thought, Lucy had underlying anxieties preventing her from demonstrating any emotions. I knew not to be judgmental, but her next visit was a real eye-opener.

This time, Lucy came without Kevin who was attending an important out-of-town meeting. She was a completely different person. Not only did she ask intelligent questions about her pregnancy, but she was personable, witty, and pleasant. The transformation was a dramatic one. While pleased with Lucy's changes, I was now suspicious that a relationship problem exited between her and Kevin;, but how to ask remained a delicate matter. I waited for the right opportunity.

"Lucy," I said calmly, "every relationship goes through times of problems." I paused to see if she had any reaction, but she continued to stare. "Are there any differences between you and Kevin?"

Lucy swallowed and didn't respond. I didn't know if I hit a raw nerve or if she was insulted by my question. She wet her lips before speaking.

"No ... no, not at all, Doctor. Why do you ask?"

Honesty is my policy, but I didn't want to offend her.

"Lucy, I hope I've said nothing to insult you, but you're a very different person today than in previous visits."

"Oh," she said with a smile. "Well, Kevin likes to run things so I let him. We're fine." She lowered her head and didn't make eye contact. "He doesn't like me to say a lot when he's around, so I don't."

Lucy had the right to remain submissive when her husband was present, but as her physician, I had the moral obligation to explore the possibility of an abusive relationship. Not only was Lucy my patient, but so was her baby. I wasn't comfortable with her response, but I hoped Lucy knew she could talk to me if needed.

In the last trimester, prenatal visits become more frequent. Lucy's personality was different depending whether Kevin was present or not. Lucy never made reference to our conversation about Kevin and remained out-going when she came to the office alone. There were no obvious signs of problems between the couple. I began to question my original concerns until early one Sunday morning, around two o'clock, when I received a call from the emergency room.

"We've got a patient of yours who is thirty-seven weeks pregnant with an injury to her abdomen and head," the ER doctor said in a perfunctory tone. "I got fetal heart tones at one hundred sixty beats per minute and no obvious internal injuries. But we need you to see her." He gave me her name.

I tried to clear my sleepy mind from the interruption. "What was the cause of the injuries?" I assumed either a car or home accident.

He paused before answering. "Well, I'm not exactly sure, but she looks scared and her mother brought her in."

Now it was registering and I asked one more question. "Is the patient's husband there?"

"No, he's not," he said. "And maybe he shouldn't be."

When I arrived in the ER, Lucy was indeed frightened but relieved to see me. She had a bruise above her right eye and on her abdomen as well. An ultrasound revealed no obvious placental injuries and the baby's heartbeat on the fetal monitor was strong with a tracing indicating fetal well-being. I spoke to her when her mother left the room. At first, she was reluctant to talk, but after a few specific questions about her injuries, she admitted that Kevin hit her several times. No, he had never done so before, although, at times, Lucy thought he might harm her. Kevin came home inebriated and an argument ensued. After hitting her, he left the house. That's when Lucy feared the baby might be injured and called her mother who insisted she be evaluated at the hospital.

On rounds the next day, Lucy seemed better. But when I brought up the subject of domestic violence, her concerns of the night before had been allayed by a phone call from Kevin.

"Oh, doctor. I'm quite all right," she said with renewed cheerfulness. "I'm sorry you had to get up in the middle of night. Kevin had a very stressful week and I shouldn't have made him so angry."

It was now apparent that the "honeymoon phase" was in effect, but I persisted to talk to her about the dangers of domestic violence, how she and her husband should seek counseling, and the need to have an exit plan in case she was exposed to another potentially violent incident. Lucy didn't seem concerned about future conflicts and wanted to go home, but I had my own serious doubts about the health of their relationship.

Kevin came to the next prenatal visit. While neither brought up the subject of that weekend incident, I felt a need to approach it again. Quickly, Kevin answered for both of them and said it was a "silly thing that happened" and that he and Lucy were fine and counseling was not necessary. I hoped they had reconciled their problems; but deep down, I knew the statistics were against a quick resolution.

Lucy's pregnancy progressed well, and at thirty-nine weeks of gestation, she went into spontaneous labor. Kevin and her mother were present and after a long labor, Lucy delivered a healthy little boy. Her postpartum period was uneventful and she looked well at her first postnatal visit without Kevin's presence. Lucy was herself again—bright, cheerful, witty, and proud of her handsome little son. But when I asked her his name, she replied "Kevin" after her husband, although she favored the name Christopher. I hoped this didn't portend future conflicts.

About six months later, Lucy called our office for a referral to a counselor. Apparently, after one of his drinking spells, Kevin hit her again. This time, Lucy sustained a facial bruise and a broken finger that didn't require surgery. Kevin agreed to therapy, but later, I discovered that he did so to appease Lucy's anger. After two sessions, Kevin refused to continue and thought it was a waste of money. While at the second session, Kevin admitted he had been "beaten up" several times as a young child by his dad and witnessed several incidents where his father physically abused his mother. Fortunately, Lucy continued to see the counselor for her own therapy, although without Kevin's permission or knowledge. Since Lucy was given a small allowance from Kevin who demanded that she account for all her expenses, her mother paid for the therapy. While Lucy wanted the relationship to work, she now recognized an additional risk—the possibility of her son being physically abused. Medical studies indicate a significant percentage of child abuse within families when there is abuse of adults.

Lucy and her therapist developed an exit plan—a method for Lucy to leave the house with her son if Kevin was to go into one of his rages. Confiding in her next-door neighbor, Lucy gave her a bag packed with necessary items including cash, a credit card her mother obtained for her, extra clothes for her and Kevin, Jr., one of his familiar toys, and both of their birth certificates. It was hard for Lucy to include her neighbor, but knew it had to be done. Lucy kept the community women's shelter's phone number in the bag as well.

Lucy left her husband and her home one night when Kevin's violence was at its worst. Again, a night of heavy drinking followed by an argument resulted in multiple injuries to Lucy. Kevin hit and kicked her repeatedly. His rage, unfortunately, extended to his 14 month-old son who woke up in fear to the sounds of screams and shouts. Kevin responded to the little boy's crying by taking him out of his crib and throwing him to the floor.

Even though drunk and violent, Kevin didn't go any further. He stormed out of the house and drove away. Lucy gathered her wits after attending to her son, called the police, went to the neighbor's house, and called the shelter. The social worker took Lucy to the ER where she was treated and released with multiple bruises and two fractured ribs. Little Kevin was emotionally traumatized and sustained a small bruise to his left shoulder.

After a police officer saw Kevin's car swerving between lanes on a major thoroughfare, he was pulled over and arrested for driving while intoxicated. At the police station, he was identified as the reported abuser. Kevin spent the night in jail but was released after one of his buddies posted bail. He immediately went to Lucy's mother's house looking for his wife and son. Lucy's mother was prepared and called the police while Kevin banged on her front door, yelling and cursing. Before the police arrived, Kevin left and later moved to an unknown place. After a few days, Lucy left the shelter and moved in with her mother, fearful that Kevin might return.

Lucy began divorce proceedings, but never saw Kevin again. A year later, she received a tearful phone call from Kevin's mother who informed her that Kevin was murdered by the jealous ex-boyfriend of a woman he was living with. Lucy's emotions were a mixture of sadness and relief. She knew it would take time for her to heal.

Lucy continued with therapy and made excellent progress. She and her son moved into an apartment and she enjoyed her new job. Her mother stayed with little Kevin during the day, and slowly, Lucy's life began to have meaning again—a life free of fear from emotional or physical abuse. She grieved for what she lost—a marriage, traditional family, and her beloved home. But Lucy also knew she was fortunate and gave back by volunteering as a counselor at the women's shelter on the weekends.

Faithfully, Lucy came to her annual gynecological visits. Her confidence and self-esteem grew significantly and Kevin, Jr., became a well-adjusted little boy. One year, Lucy inquired about birth control. She was dating a man who treated her with respect and kindness as well as adoration for little Kevin. I was happy for

Lucy—she had survived a heinous situation and now was thriving in her new life. Sadly, we both knew that her success represented a small number of those who are able to free themselves from an egregious, but unfortunately, common social affliction.

# Chapter 9

# Alice

WITH EVERY HEALTHY BABY BORN, there are obstetrical "failures" that parallel the successes—spontaneous miscarriages, fetal demises, premature births, and congenital defects. While it was more common to witness joyous reactions—the proud parents of a healthy newborn—the sadness, disappointment, and visceral sorrow for those who experienced a fetal loss remains a more powerful memory. Dealing with their emotions, as well as my own inner torment, was the most unpleasant aspect of my career as an obstetrician.

Most fetal losses are due to spontaneous errors of genetics, a somewhat comforting fact mitigating the pain of grieving parents, while others result from poor prenatal attention or to destructive habits such as smoking, drug abuse, or drinking. Yet there are fetal losses resulting from maternal illnesses, diseases that adversely affect the pregnant mother as well as her unborn fetus.

Alice was a pediatric nurse. She was a young, attractive, and bright twenty-seven-year-old who desperately wanted her own child. Alice and her husband postponed starting a family for the first two years of their marriage. While most couples wait for financial or career reasons, Alice was recommended by her internist not to conceive yet. She suffered from systemic lupus erythematosus, SLE, or lupus, a chronic inflammatory autoimmune disease affecting many different organ systems. Today, great medical strides have been made in the treatment of patients with lupus, and many live long and healthy lives with minimal problems during pregnancies. But when I began practice, the lupus patient posed a significant concern, especially if she suffered from kidney disease.

Alice's chronic lupus had caused a reduction in her kidney function. As long as she took steroids, her disease was held in check. A pregnancy could exacerbate the disease and carried a higher risk for fetal loss. If a lupus patient was in remission for more than six months prior to conception, there was a 35% risk that the disease could worsen, but a better than 90% chance of having a successful pregnancy outcome. Those patients not in remission prior to pregnancy had a much poorer prognosis with an almost fifty percent chance of further deterioration from their condition and a lower fetal survival rate. Every time Alice seemed to be on the road to remission, her lupus would "flare up" and she would postpone becoming pregnant. Against her doctor's recommendations, Alice and her husband, Rodney, decided to take a chance, and gamble that the odds would be in their favor.

Alice came to my office when she was eight weeks pregnant. Other than the usual first trimester nausea, breast tenderness, and tiredness, she looked well and had a normal blood pressure, but an urinalysis revealed a significant amount of protein. Her internist, Dr. Jon Appel, was a thorough physician but a man of few words.

"She may be stable now," he said with a reprimanding tone, "but I have some major concerns. Her renal function has slowly, but steadily decreased over the last two years, and I strongly advised her not to conceive."

"I'll follow her very closely," I said in an upbeat tone, but I knew he was convinced that, as an obstetrician, I couldn't possibly protect Alice from the dangerous mix of pregnancy and her unstable lupus condition.

My ability to monitor Alice's pregnancy was limited by the availability of technology at this time in my career. While fetal monitoring and ultrasounds were commonly used, the sophistication of obstetrical screening and prenatal evaluations did not compare to today's standards. Later on in her pregnancy, Dr. Appel informed me of a more serious concern.

"The latest blood tests were positive for antiphospholipid antibodies," he said somberly. "Like I'd told Alice before, becoming pregnant was not a good idea."

I knew what this meant. Alice had antibodies that could adversely affect her pregnancy. An antiphospholipid antibody syndrome was associated with recurrent miscarriage, poor fetal growth, and the potential for significant pregnancy induced hypertension. While progress in treating this additional autoimmune problem has improved over the years, Alice faced an almost ninety percent chance of losing the pregnancy. Significant vascular impairment of the placenta leading to early fetal demise was the rule and not the exception.

I discussed all the potential complications with Alice in a way I felt was compassionate and supportive.

"I'm aware of this condition," Alice said with a determined look. "My husband and I read about everything before we attempted conception." She swallowed. "But, we accept what could go wrong." She glanced down towards the floor. "I admit that we're both scared, but this is what we want."

Since this was before the Internet, I was impressed with Alice's desire to learn all she could. I reassured her that Dr. Appel and I would do our best to monitor her and her baby, and I knew she would be compliant with prenatal visits. Alice was given the option of seeing a "high risk" obstetrician, but she preferred to stay at our hospital.

"Doctor, what is meant to be will happen," she said confidently. Her attitude was admirable, but my concerns remained real and disturbing.

The first three months of her pregnancy were uneventful. Alice's blood pressure remained normal and the protein in her urine unchanged. Dr. Appel followed her lab tests on a consistent basis and found no evidence of progression of her disease. Fetal heart tones were easily heard and the baby appeared to be the appropriate growth on ultrasound. Not surprising, Alice and Rodney were different from most parents when hearing the heart tones, remaining reserved as well as guarded with their emotions. While Alice didn't show anxiety, I knew she felt it.

At sixteen weeks of pregnancy, Alice came to the office without complaints. But this time her blood pressure was elevated and there was more protein in her urine. The baby's heart tones were present and strong. I called Dr. Appel.

"Her renal function has decreased," he said gravely. "We may be approaching some stormy weather here."

But there was little I could do about it. I remembered Alice's comment during her first prenatal visit—"What is meant to be will happen." I recommended weekly visits.

At eighteen weeks, her blood pressure was higher and her urine protein was 4+, the highest it could be when checked by urine dipstick. Dr. Appel strongly recommended admission. Alice agreed to the hospitalization.

Her renal function deteriorated and her blood pressure continued to elevate at an alarming rate. Steroid treatment and antihypertensive drugs had minimal affect on her illness. While fetal heart tones were present, I knew placental function was affected by the exacerbation of her disease. Fetal size was no longer appropriate for her gestational dates and the placenta appeared small by ultrasound assessment. At twenty weeks and two days of gestation, no heart tones were audible and a sonogram confirmed a fetal death. Alice went into spontaneous labor and delivered a severely growth-retarded stillborn. The pathologic analysis of the placenta revealed severe vascular deterioration and compromise. Fortunately, Alice's lupus did not deteriorate during her postnatal period. Instead, her blood pressure stabilized and, after several weeks, her renal function returned to its prenatal level.

Alice and her husband were devastated, but supported each other psychologically. On her last postpartum visit, Alice expressed her appreciation for the care provided by Dr. Appel, the hospital staff, and myself. Emotionally, she remained strong and focused about the future. But all pregnancy losses were nightmares and upset me. Intellectually, I knew I did all I could and had appropriately informed Alice of the intrinsic risks of pregnancy while her lupus was active, but mentally, I felt like I had failed my patient.

Life goes on, but sometimes too quickly. Alice returned to my office for a visit four months later for what I thought would be a gynecological problem—but she was pregnant again.

"I know all the possibilities and risks," she said, eyes direct and clear. "Rodney and I know it seems unreasonable to become pregnant again so soon. Besides, we're still grieving over our loss, but we wanted to try again." Certainly, her fertility was not compromised by her illness. But I was flabbergasted by her decision to become pregnant again and so soon. When I called Dr. Appel, he responded with several seconds of silence and then a low, slow whistle. Words were not necessary.

As in the first pregnancy, Alice and her viable baby progressed on schedule until the twenty-second week of pregnancy before the same clinical features developed—severely elevated blood pressure, increased urinary protein, and ultimately, another fetal demise and delivery of a stillborn. This time, there was little to say to Alice and her husband. The memory of her previous pregnancy loss was still fresh and painful.

When I saw Alice for her last postnatal visit, her attitude changed. She talked about contraception, time to think and heal, and maybe adoption—all healthy thoughts. But seven months later, much to my dismay, Alice returned pregnant once again.

"I know you think we're crazy, but we just have a feeling this one will be okay," she said with little enthusiasm. "You don't have to inform me of the risks ... I knew them the first time, the second time, and I certainly know them now. If we lose this baby, then Rodney and I will not try ever again."

I began to question if Alice and her husband were mentally stable—a young woman with active lupus, antiphospholipid antibody syndrome, and two previous mid-trimester pregnancy losses. Was it really worth the risk to her health? But Alice's determination was undaunted. "What is meant to be will happen," she repeated again.

Emotionally, I prepared myself for the same outcome. But, surprisingly, at around twenty weeks of pregnancy, Alice didn't demonstrate any of the previous clinical signs or deterioration of her lupus condition. The fetus was developing appropriately. At twenty-seven weeks of gestation, I started getting excited. Only Dr. Appel remained skeptical and pessimistic.

"She's not out of the woods yet," he said, admonishing me for my optimism.

"I know, Jon," I replied. "But she made it to the third trimester!"

"Maybe so ... but her disease is bad; she could still end up with a stillborn, and her illness may deteriorate after her delivery," he said with an obviously annoyed tone. "She should have listened to me and not gotten pregnant again."

I knew what he said was realistic, but Alice had made it further in this pregnancy than in the last two. Her words echoed in my head. "What is meant to be will happen."

At thirty-three weeks of gestation, Alice's blood pressure became high and the protein level increased in her urine. The ultrasound revealed possible intrauterine growth retardation and a small placenta. Options were discussed, and Alice agreed to receive steroids in order to accelerate the maturation of the baby's lungs. Labor induction was begun and Alice delivered a small, but healthy boy without any problems secondary to his premature status. As before, Alice didn't have any deterioration to her lupus after delivery. She and Rodney were ecstatic. I was as well, and much relieved about the good outcome. While she had gambled with odds significantly against her, Alice and her husband had won—and their payoff was a healthy child. I knew Alice would be a caring and conscientious mother.

Alice's successful pregnancy outcome would remain a highlight in my medical career, but I didn't anticipate the next stage to her tumultuous medical history. About nine months later, I received a call from the hospital for a consultation. Alice was in the ICU with severe deterioration of her lupus condition. Dr. Appel asked me to be notified. I did not recognize her when I went to the bedside. Where was the young healthy woman I had seen at her six-week postpartum visit? Alice was on a respirator, her face swollen beyond recognition, and a catheter in her bladder produced bloody urine. I reviewed her chart and read Dr. Appel's finely written penmanship. Alice was in a lupus flare-up severely affecting her kidneys, heart, brain, and blood count. I cringed when I read his prognosis—her condition was grave and he doubted survival. One morning when I went to visit her, another patient was in the room. The nurse informed me that Alice had died during the night.

Although I was prepared intellectually, I wasn't emotionally. I stared out the window, deeply distraught. Alice's nurse sat next to me, anticipating my shock.

"She was a strong and wonderful woman," she said, eyes moist with tears. "We'll miss her as a friend and colleague."

"Yes," I mumbled.

She sighed. "You know, we knew a few days ago Alice wasn't going to make it. But, all of us, including the nurses and the staff, couldn't believe Dr. Appel's reaction when he came in to pronounce her death. We'd never have guessed it."

I turned towards her, eyes wide. "What do you mean by his reaction?"

"Well," she said with head lowered. "Dr. Appel just wept uncontrollably as he wrote his notes."

I had underestimated the emotions of Alice's internist. While apparently cool and detached with his tough persona, Dr. Appel fooled us all. Today, when we pass in the hospital hallways, he remains aloof and reserved. But, I know that there is another side to him, one of compassion with more emotional energy than he is willing to expose.

I never heard what happened to Alice's husband and her child, but I hope there is a young man in this world who has been told over and over about his determined and courageous mother, even though he may not remember her. And when he's facing a difficult situation in life, I hope he will think or say, "What is meant to be will happen."

## CHAPTER 10

# Laura

DURING MOST FIRST PRENATAL VISITS, I have the opportunity to explore more than medical issues—the patient's perspective and knowledge about pregnancy, labor and delivery, child rearing, and the relationship with her partner as well as her own personal maturity. Some were easy to read—from the young couple excited about their new adventure to the unmarried adolescent with the mind of a child within an adult's body. Other patients were more difficult to assess initially, but with time and trust, would reveal their inner selves and expectations. Laura's first visit was more than revealing, a unique situation that began with tragedy and ended with determined courage.

Every new patient interview begins with the necessary medical history, followed by questions about social and emotional issues. Laura moved to Houston from upstate New York just three months before she conceived for the first time. She was healthy, didn't smoke or drink, and appeared poised and pleasant. But I didn't expect the response to one of my questions.

"Does your husband want to be in the delivery room when you go into labor?" I asked as a routine entry into the non-medical, although equally as important personal history.

Laura's countenance changed suddenly as she lowered her head. Quickly, I tightened my mouth as I glanced at the patient information sheet listing specifics including marital status, angry with myself for not checking it before asking this question. I expected to see "single" or "divorced," but instead, Laura had written "married." Why did she respond this way?

Laura raised her head and stared at me, focused and resolved, an image still vivid within my memory. Her eyes were moist from suppressed tears. What was I missing?

"My husband died three weeks ago," she said, words barely audible.

I swallowed. "I'm, oh, I'm so sorry," I said sincerely. Laura's response caught me off-guard and I needed a few seconds to regain my thoughts.

I leaned back in my chair. "Do you have any family here?"

"No," she said with a sigh.

I twisted my lips. "Any family back in Rochester?"

Laura slowly shook her head. "No. My father died when I was little and my mom died two years ago. I have two cousins who live in Syracuse, but I haven't spoken to them in several years."

I maintained my professionalism, but from deep inside, I felt great sympathy as well as pity for Laura—a new place, pregnancy, and now, no husband. Not only did I wonder how she was going to make it emotionally without a partner, family, or friends, but I was concerned about her husband's death as well—illness, trauma, suicide?

Laura never volunteered anything further about the circumstances of her husband's death during that first visit. When I asked about her emotional state, she smiled and assured me she was fine. I continued with the rest of the history, performed an exam and Pap smear, and obtained the prenatal blood panel. Laura was given an appointment for the following month. That evening, I carried Laura's situation home with me. How could this young person keep her composure and focus on her pregnancy? But I didn't know how strong she was yet.

Laura's prenatal visits were problem free. She became excited about the pregnancy, never bringing up the subject of her deceased husband. Most obstetrical patients required a great deal of counseling during their visits—questions about their physical changes, anxieties about labor and delivery, the baby, and concerns about the hospital staff, maternity unit, and pediatrician. With Laura, every visit was quick and routine. Her questions were minimal but always appropriate and she never appeared confused, tense, or depressed. She came to visits alone—no friends or extended family.

At thirty-nine weeks of gestation, Laura went into labor and drove herself to the hospital. Her vital signs were normal and the fetal monitor indicated well-being. Laura was determined to have the baby naturally, without any anesthetic, even though her labor progressed slowly with strong and painful contractions. After seven hours and minimal dilation of the cervix, I spoke to Laura as her doctor and, perhaps because of her unusual circumstances, as a friend as well.

"Laura," I said as calmly as possible. "I know you told me you don't want an anesthetic, but you're making minimal progress and I'm concerned you may become too fatigued. Why don't you agree to an epidural anesthetic? It'll give you pain relief and allow you to rest and possibly help you progress quicker?"

She stared at the ceiling while using her Lamaze techniques. Not once did she ask for any pain medication. When her contraction began to decrease, she spoke. "No, I don't want an anesthetic." Her words were weak and unconvincing.

"Why?" I asked incredulously. She was healthy and had no contraindications to an epidural anesthetic. Her resistance was inconsistent with her usual common sense and intelligence observed during her prenatal visits.

Laura began another contraction. This one seemed particularly long and painful. When it ended, she gazed at me with tearful eyes.

"I'm scared!" she said as she shook her head. I held her sweaty hand and wondered why. The reason soon became apparent.

"Laura, what frightens you about an anesthetic?"

She swallowed and wet her lips. "My husband," she said, her voice trembling. "He died from an anesthetic during a routine gall bladder operation." She turned her head away from me and sobbed.

Now it was clear. Although anesthetic complications are rare, I had a hunch about what may have happened to her husband. I waited until the next contraction finished.

"Laura," I said softly, "did your husband die from a condition called malignant hyperthermia?"

Her eyes widened. "Yes. That what the doctors told me." She took a deep breath. "We didn't know of any one in his family with this condition." She sighed. "The doctors were all so good. They did everything they could, but the damage was too much."

Malignant hyperthermia is a rare genetic disease. When the patient is exposed to certain drugs, anesthetics, or extreme heat, it can set off a chain of events, including muscle damage, kidney, and heart failure. While extremely rare, it is preventable if there is knowledge of a family history for the disease or it is diagnosed before one of these events occur. Most cases of malignant hyperthermia are treatable at the time of the incident, but apparently, in Laura's husband's case, the insults were too quick and damaging—a most unfortunate and rare tragedy. Today, the anesthetic agents used are different when Laura was in labor. Now was the time for me to teach, guide, and support my patient.

"Laura, I understand why you're so adamantly against an anesthetic. But I want to reassure you that your husband's reaction to the anesthetic was an extremely rare event, and doesn't occur during an epidural anesthetic."

She blinked. "It doesn't?"

"No. And it might help you relax so that your labor can progress. And if you should require a cesarean section, then we can use the epidural for that procedure."

Another long and hard contraction. When it was over, she looked at me with her usual focused expression.

"Okay," she said. "I believe you. And, I guess I should have told you this before I went into labor. But, I didn't want to think about it and I hoped I could deliver vaginally without any anesthetic or pain medication."

I held her hand during another contraction. When it was over, I found her nurse and asked her to call the anesthesiologist. When he arrived, I explained the situation to him, and he reassured Laura just as I had done. Twenty-five minutes later, Laura was free of labor pain.

Laura progressed after her epidural and about three hours later gave birth to a healthy boy. On rounds the next day, I arrived in Laura's room while she was breast feeding her new son.

"What a handsome and healthy boy you have there!" I said sincerely.

"Yes," she said staring at her new baby with the inimitable look of a new mother's love.

"What's his name?" I asked.

Laura paused. She smiled at her son and looked at me, tears running down her cheeks.

"I named him after my husband," she said with a whisper. "He was born on his birthday."

I don't remember what I said, but I do recall leaving the hospital in a daze. Later that evening, I tried to read one of the many medical journals stacked on my desk at home, but I kept thinking about what Laura said. I felt that something miraculous occurred with the birth of her child. This was, in the truest sense, Laura's spiritual birthday gift to her deceased husband. And I had the privilege of witnessing it.

Laura has continued to see me for her gynecological care for the past twenty-five years and is proud of her son who is a healthy and successful young adult. While we never chat about her past, I know there's a special memory we will share about a most singular and extraordinary event.

# PART VI

# Adulthood

# CHAPTER 11

# Cathy

Ever since I stopped delivering babies, it's unusual to be awakened by a phone call after midnight; but one night, the annoying ring of the phone startled me from a deep and peaceful sleep. Before I made my decision to quit maternity, I received a call from a colleague's patient at four in the morning. A nineteen-year-old, worried about her first pregnancy, called with what she thought was an obstetrical emergency. When the answering service connected me, the patient spoke sobbed between words. Quickly, I sat up in my bed prepared for a medical disaster.

"Please try to settle down ma'am," I said with concern. "I can't understand what you're saying."

Slowly, she gained composure. "I think I just lost my mucous plug!"

My lips tightened as I forced myself to suppress what I thought was the appropriate response—"Well, what do you want me to do? Help you find it?"

Fortunately, I held my tongue, but this proved to be the *coup de grace*—my cynical attitude was uncharacteristic, and I knew the strain of obstetrics was the cause. Although I miss that special moment when parents bond with their newborn, I have never regretted quitting maternity and specializing in gynecological surgery. While problems arise with post-op patients necessitating sleepy-time interruptions, most calls are not urgent in nature. Unless it is a true emergency, I can settle down quickly and go back to sleep (something I have perfected well over the years). But this night, the three-AM phone call not only disrupted my sleep but created a proverbial nightmare.

A general surgery colleague, Dr. Steven Wilson, was calling from the emergency room. One of my gynecological patients was in the ER with a two-day history of right-sided abdominal pain, fever, nausea, and vomiting. The consulting general surgeon suspected a ruptured appendix, but a CAT scan, ordered by the ER doctor, revealed the possibility of a right ovarian mass with free fluid in the abdomen and pelvis.

"You know, I still think it's her appendix," the surgeon said, "but this damn scan has got me confused and I would rather have you here just in case."

I knew the doctor well, and while he could be a bit earthy and crass with his language and mannerisms, he was a gifted technician with a big, warm and friendly heart. His clinical expertise was irreproachable.

"Okay," I said trying to sound awake even though I knew I was failing, "give me fifteen minutes."

During my drive to the hospital, I had time to think about the patient. Although I don't recall everyone, usually I can match a patient's name with her face as well as the medical history. Cathy became my patient several years before. After an emotionally draining divorce, she found a decent job in Houston and moved from her home in Pittsburgh. She had two daughters; one was a freshman at Boston University and the other a sophomore in high school who was happy to move with her mother to a new town with a warm climate. The two settled in well, and the daughter easily made new friends. She did well in high school and was currently a junior at Texas Tech University. Cathy was an affable forty-seven-year-old, a responsible mother with a great sense of humor and strong work ethics, but she was unsuccessful at healthy relationships. When she came for her yearly visits, she complained how difficult it was to meet "good" men among all the "losers" out "there." While I couldn't give Cathy relationship counseling, I tried to support her emotionally. Cathy had no history of gynecological problems. The general surgeon is probably right I thought—it must be a ruptured appendix involving the right ovary. Hopefully, the surgery would be quick and easy and I would be back in my comfortable bed, sleeping soundly.

The uncomfortable glare from the florescent lights seemed brighter at night, and I winced when entering the pre-op suite. Instead of the upbeat and amiable person I knew, Cathy moaned as she lay in the fetal position. Her pulse rate was rapid and her forehead sweaty. The nurses' notes listed her temperature at 103.6 degrees and the white blood cell was elevated. Cathy could barely talk, and I didn't have the heart to lay my hands on her tender and swollen belly.

She was able to respond to some of my questions and denied any menstrual problems since her last visit. I explained the CAT scan findings and our working diagnosis of a ruptured appendix. If any gynecological problems were found, I told her, I would need to do what was surgically indicated. She nodded while groaning, eyes tightly closed with strands of tears slowly running down her cheeks. I gently rubbed her back and left to change into surgical scrubs.

Cathy was taken to the OR, given a general anesthetic, and prepared for the exploratory laparotomy. I scrubbed my hands, and found the strong plastic smell from my surgical mask unpleasant. Dr. Wilson was silent as we shared the sink, probably exhausted from other emergency surgeries earlier in the evening. We entered the OR room and took our places along the table. As he made the incision across Cathy's lower abdomen, I felt a gradual heightened tension in anticipation of the findings. Slowly, we opened the last layer of the abdominal wall, the peritoneum, moments away from seeing the insides of the human body.

"Wowee!" Dr. Wilson shouted. "What in the world is going on here?"

Copious amount of pus spewed out. I knew this was too much for a ruptured appendix. Whatever type of infectious process fulminated in Cathy's abdomen, it was severe and at best would cause a stormy post-op course. We suctioned the pus out, obtaining appropriate cultures and continued to explore Cathy's insides.

It didn't take long to find the source. Cathy had a ruptured abscess on her right tube and ovary. The entire pelvis, uterus, and the other tube and ovary were involved as well. The appendix and several loops of bowel were wrapped around the complex collection of pus. Our anesthesiologist, a crusty curmudgeon with good clinical instincts, started the appropriate fluids and antibiotics hoping to reduce the risk of a bacterial sepsis, or blood infection, a condition that could be life threatening. Quickly, Dr. Wilson and I began our surgical challenge by removing of the uterus, tubes, ovaries, and appendix.

Fortunately, we were able to free the loops of bowel from the infected mass without resecting these organs. But, the infected tissues bled easily because of the significant inflammatory process, and Cathy needed to be transfused with several units of blood. Dr. Wilson and I worked well together, saying little, and putting all our efforts into a difficult surgery with a high risk for complications and injury. After three hours of intense concentration, we closed her abdominal after placement of several drains. I was exhausted, but I knew I needed to remain alert and vigilant for a rough postoperative course.

Cathy did well with the anesthetic, thanks to our no-nonsense anesthesiologist. Her vital signs remained stable throughout the surgery, lungs ventilated well, and urine output was adequate. The morning nursing shift began to arrive for work. The freshly brewed coffee aroma smelled wonderfully delicious and I realized I was hungry, common after operating for several hours. As I entered the staff room, I met one of my patients, a recovery room nurse, just coming on duty.

"My, oh my," she said with a smile, "didn't expect to see you here this morning."

"Shelley," I said. "This was a bad one ... a ruptured tubo-ovarian abscess. Do you mind taking care of her?"

"No, not at all," she said confidently. I knew her medical skills were good and felt some reassurance with her as Cathy's recovery room nurse. I drank the coffee and went to the surgical waiting room. No family members were present, only Cathy's neighbor, also a patient of mine. I told her Cathy was stable and asked if she knew anything more.

"No, not really," she said. "Cathy called me yesterday and complained about a fever and stomach pain. She had some antibiotics left over from a bladder infection from several months ago and took them. But she called me at around ten last night sounding very sick, so I brought her to the ER."

Her friend was exhausted from a fitful sleep in a chair. I told her to go home, call Cathy's daughters, and get some rest.

I went back into the recovery room to check Cathy again. Her blood pressure and urine output looked good. How many insults can one body take?, I thought. Sometimes it's not the great new technology or the advanced drugs that heal a patient, but the constitution and the internal milieu of one's anatomy, physiology, and other non-defined elements, an intrinsic reserve not defined by scientific terminology, separating the "saved" from the "deaths."

With Shelley attending the patient, I felt comfortable enough to go home and get some rest. After a full breakfast and a little bit of time to "come down" from the night's activities, I fell asleep. Three hours later, the phone rang. It was Shelley.

"I'm not sure what's going on, but Cathy's got a temperature of 104.6. Her blood count is good, but her white count is extremely low, kidney function slightly decreased, and liver function tests a bit out of whack." I knew her well enough to hear the concern in her voice.

I asked Shelley to page Dr. John Regan, an excellent internist with additional training in infectious diseases. I knew we had problems. Cathy's clinical presentation was suggestive of sepsis or a blood infection. I knew I couldn't manage her condition without further help.

Dr. Regan was already there when I arrived, a hard-working doctor who practically lived at the hospital. He was either walking in the hallways or his name was being incessantly paged over the speakers. I found him sitting at the nurses' station writing notes in Cathy's chart, stethoscope wrapped around his neck and index cards stuffed into every pocket of his white coat.

"John," I asked anxiously. "What do you think?" Much to my surprise, he appeared unnerved by Cathy's clinical situation.

"Oh, I think she'll be fine. You have her on the right antibiotics, which we can change if the cultures reveal any resistance, and her vital signs and urine output are stable." He yawned.

Maybe because I take care of healthy patients while Dr. Regan tends to the very sick, I was surprised by his composure. Cathy's liver, as well as her kidneys, was probably infected with bacteria from the pelvic abscess. How could he be so nonchalant?

"She had major insult from the infection and surgery coupled with blood loss," he said calmly. "But, she has no previous medical problems." He leaned back in his chair and took a sip of coffee. "Maybe a few rough days, but she'll be all right."

I swallowed and wished I could be less anxious, but this was my patient who was ill and remained my emotional burden.

Cathy went to the surgical ICU. I thanked Shelley for her good nursing care. The ICU clerk informed me that one of Cathy's daughters was in the waiting room. Julie looked scared and tired. While Lubbock is in the same state, Houston is almost a nine-hour drive from her university dormitory. She left as soon as the neighbor, Sally, called her, stopping only once to use the restroom, and made it in less than eight hours. Julie was a perceptive young woman, and while I tried to assuage her apprehension, I knew she could detect my own concerns.

"Doctor?" she asked, tears welling in her eyes, "should I call my sister Megan to fly down here?" Her older sister graduated from college and was living and working in Washington, D.C.

I shook my head. "No, not now." I put my hand on her shoulder. "Just call and tell her we'll keep her up to date."

I brought her into the ICU and knew that the sight of her mother hooked up to noisy monitors, large IV machines, a bladder catheter, and several abdominal drains pooling blood tinged fluid would be unsettling. I felt terrible for Julie—she was alone without the presence of her father or sister. She agreed to go home, try to collect her feelings, get some rest, and return in a few hours.

I went home myself. But I called the ICU almost every two hours. Nothing changed with Cathy's condition. That night, as tired as I was, I slept restlessly. On Monday morning, I awoke physically and emotionally drained. But I had a full day of patients and I was anxious to see Cathy. On my drive to the hospital, I hoped to find her sitting up in bed, smiling and feeling well. I pushed the automatic door opener and entered the ICU, a hectic scene with doctors, nurses, respiratory therapists, and clerks busy tending to the sickest patients in the hospital. I found Cathy's nurse who was preparing a patient for the OR. She informed me that Cathy's vital signs and urine output remained stable, but her kidney and liver function was worse. A cold sweat formed on the back of my neck and I paged Dr. Regan.

"Hey, don't be so worried," he said cheerfully. "I've already checked on her and I still think she'll be fine."

His comment did little to reassure me. At lunchtime, I went to the ICU again and found Cathy no different. When I finished with office patients around six, I went back, hoping by now Cathy would be significantly improved.

Her ICU nurse was busy again with another sick patient, and I'm sure she thought Cathy was the least of her problems.

"She's the same doc. No better, no worse," she said while putting a second IV into her patient.

Slowly, I walked to Cathy's room and found Julie at her bedside, rubbing her mother's back. She looked at me, eyes wide and fearful.

"She's breathing so hard," she said. "What's wrong with her lungs?"

Lungs, I thought? Yes, Cathy's respiration rate was faster than earlier. While her monitor indicated an acceptable blood oxygen level, clinically, I knew something was not right. I ordered arterial blood gases and a chest x-ray. When I received the results, I swallowed hard and paged Dr. Regan. I knew enough internal medicine to make the diagnosis—Cathy was in acute respiratory distress syndrome or ARDS for short.

ARDS is a serious lung disease resulting from any bodily insult, such as trauma, toxic inhalation, near drowning, and most frequently, from a severe infection. The mortality rate associated with ARDS is 35-40%, but may reach almost 90% after bacterial sepsis. Now my concerns were heightened and I feared for Cathy's life. Dr. Regan answered his page and came to the ICU quickly. After reviewing the new findings, he made the decision—Cathy needed mechanical ventilation. She was sedated, intubated, and hooked to a breathing machine for respiratory assistance. I stood by Cathy's bedside feeling helpless.

I let Julie back, watching her stare at her mom with one hand covering her mouth.

"Doctor," she said between sniffles. "I'm scared."

I swallowed hard and thought of euphemistic words to temper the situation. None came to mind, so I decided to treat Julie as a friend or family member rather than as the daughter of my patient.

"Julie," I said softly, "I'm scared too."

Surprised with my un-doctor like response, she nodded and seemed more at ease. By sharing my own emotions, her fears were validated and mitigated some of the intensity. Julie knew everything was being done for her mom and only time would give us an outcome. Julie kissed her mother's swollen cheek and thanked me for my help. She left to call her sister.

The next three days were a cloudy memory. I slept little, did my work and interacted with my patients as professionally as possible, and made four to five visits to the ICU per day as well as frequent phone calls to check on Cathy's condition. Julie remained strong throughout the ordeal. At night, while I'd try to fall asleep, I wondered if Cathy would be my first surgical patient to die. I questioned all I did over and over, but knew there was little else but to wait and see.

Thursday morning, I picked up the phone and called the ICU as I had for the past several days, hoping that Cathy's condition had not worsened. I was now familiar with most of the hard working ICU nurses.

"How did Cathy do last night, Jim?"

"Well, doctor," he said, "Cathy had a most eventful night."

My heart rate quickened as I jumped out of bed, feeling a wave of terror. I expected the worst news.

"Cathy pulled her tube out around two-thirty this morning. She's breathing fine on her own and her blood gases are good"

I sat back on my bed. "What? So ... so she looks better?" I stuttered.

"Yes. And her kidney and liver numbers are a heck of a lot better too."

Quickly, I showered and went in to see her. Much to my amazement, Cathy was sitting up in bed and watching TV. She didn't remember a thing. I explained all the events to her.

"Guess I've been a pain in the butt," she said with a grin. I smiled for the first time in many days.

Cathy not only got better, but quickly as well. When her kidney and liver function returned to normal a few days later, she went home. On her return visit, the clinical picture became clearer. A few nights before she became ill, Cathy met a man at a single's club and had relations with him without protection. Whatever STD she caught was mitigated by the antibiotics she took, but not enough to quell an infection brewing into a flagrant pelvic abscess with eventual rupture creating a life-threatening injury to her kidneys, liver, and lungs.

"You know, doctor," she said with her head tilted, "I've been living out that old country and Western song. You know, 'looking for love in all the wrong places.' Guess I should have known better."

Yes, I thought. We all think that we should have known better when we realize our mistakes, but when you learn from your errors, you gain maturity.

"Cathy," I said. "Why don't you try to let go a bit? You know ... let things happen and be happy with yourself."

She paused pensively and nodded. "Yes, you're right." She looked at me. "Thanks, Doc," she said smiling. "And thanks for your care as well as your advice."

When I saw her six months later, she was doing well with a few minor residual pulmonary difficulties.

"You know, Doctor, I took your advice. I stopped trying to make things happen, like finding a partner. And, believe it or not, the less I try, the more I seem to meet interesting people, good people, people I like to be around." I was pleased to hear this.

A year later, Cathy came for a routine visit. She looked great—healthy and happy. Her oldest daughter, Megan, moved to Texas, and she and Julie shared an apartment in Austin. Much to my delight, Cathy was dating a man for the past several months, a relationship that appeared mutual and healthy. I was delighted for Cathy and her family—they had all grown from a near tragic situation. As for me, when a patient's phone call wakes me in the middle of the night, I deal with it, grateful that it's a minor one.

# Chapter 12

# Jill

TODAY, MOST DOCTORS join a physician group when they complete their residency training. As a solo practitioner, I have both advantages and disadvantages. Although I own my professional association and can make all the decisions without conflict with other physicians or administrators, I have no income if I'm not working. Additionally, I am responsible for corporate details as well, but the most burdensome problem is when I'm in surgery or out of town and need to rely on other physicians to cover for emergencies. This inherent problem was resolved when I met Jill.

For many years, I have been medical director of a local Planned Parenthood clinic. My role includes availability for questions by the Planned Parenthood nurse practitioners as well as monthly chart reviews. Planned Parenthood provides preventive care and birth control counseling regardless of income, race ethnicity, sexual orientation, nationality, or residence. Patients have affordable access to a health clinic that provides compassionate and conscientious care. While the organization is maligned for providing termination services, the clinic I direct does not perform abortions, but appropriate counseling and care. Jill was a nurse practitioner for Planned Parenthood when I first met her.

After completing her nursing degree, Jill worked for the labor and delivery unit and later for the gynecology service at our hospital, but she felt she could do more as a nurse. She returned to school and after extensive clinical training, became a nurse practitioner, joined Planned Parenthood, and found her role as a nurse clinician rewarding and productive. Jill would "float" from one clinic to the next filling in for the regulars who were on vacation or at a medical meeting. When I met her at my clinic, she expressed interest in working in a private practice setting. I never considered the possibility of a nurse practitioner in my office, but it made sense.

Jill brought a new dimension to our services. Whenever I was in surgery or if my schedule was too packed for further appointments, Jill could see a patient who needed care that day. While I believe it is the physician and not the gender that makes a doctor effective as a care-provider, there were patients who preferred seeing another female—one who could treat their problems with a different sense of empathy and compassion. Jill fitted in well and was immediately accepted by the nurses and staff. She possessed the diplomacy, as well as the personality, to work as a team player.

At thirty-six years of age, Jill was healthy and a passionate runner. She was tall, 6 foot 2 inches, and a star college basketball player for a local university. Originally from southern California, she was accepted to college on an athletic as well as academic scholarship. When Jill was a senior, she met Dennis who was a MBA graduate student and an All American college football player. After marriage, they bought a home and began a family. When I met Jill, their daughters were age three and seven and Dennis was happy with his position for a large oil company. Eventually, when I got to know him, Dennis seemed amiable and generous.

While I consider my clinical observation skills to be sharp, my ability to discern differences about furniture, clothes, or the ordinary things in life are, unfortunately, blunted. One of my nurses asked to speak to me privately at the end of a busy day.

"I'm concerned about Jill," she said. "She's lost a lot of weight."

"Really," I asked, not having the faintest idea if Jill looked any different this day than the first day I met her. "How long has she appeared this way?"

"Oh, about the last few months. All the other girls agree with me."

While my staff people are not gossipers, they were worried about Jill.

"Is she training for a marathon?" I asked.

"No," my nurse said. "But she did say she was running more lately."

"Well, there you go!" I said as if the problem was resolve;, but my staff possesses that powerful insight, women's intuition, a combination of both conscious and unconscious signals, seemingly deficient or possibly completely lacking in most men.

Jill worked three days a week, so I didn't see her until after the weekend. But this time I did notice her thinness. And she appeared more tired than usual. Yet, there was no apparent compromise to her patient care and clinical decision-making. I debated to ask her if everything was all right, but decided to wait and see instead.

A few weeks later, I noticed red flags. First, Jill was an hour late to the office, unusual for her promptness. But it wasn't until I saw a patient for an unresolved problem that it became apparent something was wrong with Jill.

"Your nurse practitioner," the patient said angrily, "didn't listen to what I was telling her. She looked real spacey, like she was thinking of something else."

Now, I needed to speak to Jill. While I was troubled about Jill's problem, I was also concerned about my patients' welfare. At the end of the day, I asked her to come into my office.

Jill looked fatigued and appeared quite thin. When I asked her if anything was bothering her, she stared wide-eyed for a few moments before starting to cry. She reached for a tissue and tried to regain her composure.

"I'm sorry," she said as she shook her head. "I hoped this wouldn't affect my work."

"Jill," I said calmly as I leaned forward. "You don't have to tell me anything you don't want to. But, if I can help, please let me."

"No," she said softly, eyes gazing downward. "I thought I could handle this and keep everything quiet at the same time." She looked up. "I'm a nurse and I should know better."

For the next thirty minutes, Jill told me about her recent marital problems. When Dennis was in college, he tended to have bouts of binge drinking and one time ended up in jail for getting into a fight with a student from a rival college. Dennis came from a family with a history of alcoholism. According to Jill, Dennis was dissatisfied with his career and started drinking more on the weekends. When he missed a day's work due to a hangover, Jill said they needed to talk. She shared her concerns with Dennis, not only for his well-being but for their daughters' as well.

"He's been such a good father," she said, wiping her eyes. "He loves the girls and I know he loves me, but this drinking is ruining our family. I find bottles of booze and beer in the garbage can, in his study, and even in his car. I'm scared he'll get in an accident, or worse, kill an innocent victim."

I took a deep breath. What a shame, I thought.

"What about AA?" I asked.

Jill swallowed. "We talked about it and Dennis said he would consider it, but I'm afraid he won't go."

The problem was serious and I knew it would not be resolved soon. I needed to offer help while she and Dennis tried to work it out.

"Are you sleeping well at night?"

Jill sighed. "No, not at all. I can fall asleep easily since I'm so tired, but I wake up about three hours later and can't fall back to sleep. After the girls are in bed, I try to run a few more miles, hoping it will help me sleep better, but it never does. It's hard for me to concentrate during the day. I've lost my appetite, and sometimes, I get real nervous and panicky."

Jill's emotional and physical state had all the hallmarks of situational depression and anxiety. While there is more public awareness for depression, nearly eighty percent of cases are undiagnosed. Depressive episodes can be triggered by life events—from a loss, disability, or medical disease—as well as in the absence of any situational or psychological trauma. Many patients believe they shouldn't feel this way and that treatment is unnecessary. While a family history of depression is a risk factor, so is a history of substance abuse, physical or sexual violence, as well as the loss of a parent during childhood. Jill had none of these risks, but her stressful family situation was the obvious triggering event.

When I recommended counseling, Jill scheduled an appointment with a psychologist the following week, but Dennis refused to attend—not a good sign. I asked Jill if she needed time off, but she shook her head no.

"Do you think an antidepressant may help?"

"No," she said defiantly. "I want to do this on my own without medication."

Although this was a typical patient response, the newer generations of antidepressants, called selective serotonin reuptake inhibitors, or SSRIs (as already addressed in the story about Cindy), are safe and have revolutionized treatment for most depressive states. Without any addictive properties and with a good safety profile, these drugs help many cope with depressions. While the SSRIs don't always work and have some side effects, especially dry mouth and decreased libido, they are generally well tolerated and are effective relatively quickly.

Jill's desire to solve her problems without a medication was admirable, but at least my suggestion opened the door to possible use later. Jill was strong-minded, but I knew if her situation became worse, she would acquiesce and consider taking the medication.

Dennis did go to Alcoholics Anonymous, a huge step on his behalf. Jill attended counseling once a week, and found it helpful. In addition, Jill went to Al-Anon meetings, an organization supporting family and friends of alcoholics. Over the next several weeks, Jill began to sleep better and her appetite improved. I was happy for her. I knew the journey to recovery would be tough for Dennis, but I believed the right thing would happen.

Unfortunately, the road became rockier and eventually came to a dead end. Dennis stopped going to AA, began drinking again, missed work at least once a week, and was eventually fired from his position. Jill pleaded with him to seek counseling and return to AA. But his addiction continued, and according to Jill, he denied a problem and began blaming her for his miseries. Their older daughter began acting out at school, resulting in disciplinary problems, and her grades, usually excellent, deteriorated.

Jill became depressed and anxious again. She was able to perform her nurse practitioner duties, but continued to lose weight and remained chronically fatigued. We talked again about the use of a SSRI.

She shook her head. "No, but thanks for asking. My counseling and running are my best therapies."

But the tension at home escalated. Dennis sat in front of the TV all day and refused to look for another job. Jill's attempts to motivate him were unsuccessful, and eventually he became angry with her for not supporting him during a crisis "caused by his lousy employer." She knew she had to let Dennis find his way but wondered how long she could manage to run the house, take care of the children, earn an income, and put up with Dennis' denials. The final blow came one night.

Dennis came home at two o'clock one morning inebriated and attempted to make eggs and bacon. He dropped pots and pans during the process waking Jill from a light sleep resulting in an animated argument. Jill poured her heart out, telling Dennis that she couldn't see him self-destruct and bring their family down with him. Dennis shouted obscenities and blamed her for all his problems. The two girls were awakened by the noise and fearfully watched the altercation from the top of the stairs. Dennis, in his rage, took a frying pan and threw it at Jill, striking her right knee. When their mother went down in pain, the girls began screaming and crying. Dennis stormed out of the house and drove away. Jill was able to regain her composure and calm her hysterical daughters.

Fortunately, her knee was only bruised, but the marriage was broken. Jill felt she had no other choice but to leave with the girls. While in pain, physically and emotionally, she packed clothes and personal items and began to drive to her parent's house in Los Angeles around four AM. She was confused as well as scared.

Jill did not get any further than San Antonio when she received a call on her cell phone from the police. Dennis was arrested for driving while intoxicated and was in jail. Jill turned off her phone and thought long and hard while the two girls slept in the back seat. With tears in her eyes, she turned around and stared at her peaceful children.

"I'm sorry, girls," she whispered between sobs. "But I have to do this for our sake. Please don't ever blame me."

Jill made up her mind and headed back to Houston, but her plans didn't include posting bail for Dennis. Instead, once at home, she had the locks on the doors changed and made an appointment to see an attorney. While it hurt, intellectually she knew divorce was her best option.

The death of a relationship is like the death of a person. The emotional ups and downs reflect the usual grieving process of shock, denial, bargaining, and hopefully, acceptance, intermixed with anger, fear, guilt, and loneliness. There is no predictable process to this loss, and the emotions can change minute by minute. Jill continued to go to counseling, Al-Anon, and exercised regularly, but struggled with her fatigue and anxiety. She knew it was time.

"I've thought it over," she told me one day. "I'd like for you to prescribe an SSRI for me."

"Okay, Jill," I said. "You know the risks and complications. And I support your decision."

It took about two weeks, but Jill's sleeping pattern began to improve from two to three hours a night to five hours. By the end of the month, she was sleeping almost six hours without interruptions.

"I'm surprised," she told me one day at lunch. She was looking more rested and I noticed she was drinking bottled water instead of the never-ending coffee with the ubiquitous half-empty cups scattered throughout the office.

"I don't feel much different other than I can think clearer and I have less anxiety. Other than that, I still feel all my emotions as I did before, but I can cope with them. Thank you for your offer and particularly for your patience. I know I resisted, but this medication is helping me through a tough time in my life."

I was pleased. While not everyone responds to these drugs as well as Jill did, I knew she could focus on her problems more effectively. Jill and Dennis were divorced nine months later, and while there are those who divorce their parental responsibilities as well, Dennis' love for his children brought him out of his denial.

He went to counseling as well as AA, stopped drinking, obtained a decent position with another company, and became the dad he used to be. While not a traditional family structure, Dennis and Jill were able to raise their children within the environment of two separate homes. Unfortunately, for some divorced parents, the fight continues and children are used as weapons within their arsenal, a tragic situation. Fortunately, Jill and Dennis were able to communicate in a civil fashion about issues concerning the girls. Jill stayed on her medication for almost two years, but eventually stopped taking it without difficulty, although she was fearful that the old emotions would resurface.

What had happened to Jill made her more empathetic and understanding with patients who needed medication assistance during traumatic times. While an advocate for a healthy life style and the use of medication as a last resort, Jill was able to counsel her patients effectively as well as offering them drug options.

Every once in a while, I notice Jill at the office medicine closet taking samples of a SSRI for a patient she thinks would benefit. As a survivor of an emotionally traumatic time, Jill was able to assist those who walked in the dark through a seemingly hopeless, endless tunnel of depression.

# CHAPTER 13

# **Anna**

A MEDICAL PRACTICE is a dynamic process, from the early years creating a patient base, to a well-established clientele sustained by patient referrals, to near retirement. The evolution of a doctor's practice has many subtle, but strong, influences paralleling our own lives—economic, social, cultural, and political factors. A practice is always in a state of flux, reflecting the vicissitudes of life itself. Like our own personal journeys, there are basic tenets that allow us to adapt and survive, such as honesty, hard work, ethics, and dedication to improvement. The old adage, "the more things change, the more they stay the same," applies to everything we experience and how we view our roles in the challenges of our careers, as well as in the game of life. For me, the opportunity to observe patients "grow up"—from the anxieties of being a new young mother to the uncertainties of midlife changes—has been a privilege. Such was the case of Anna.

Like many "northerners," Anna and her husband, Patrick, moved to Houston in the late 1970s—a time of tremendous growth in the "Sun Belt" cities, contrasted with the economic depressions of the northern metropolises. While economic climates cycle, Houston provided career opportunities within a good environment for raising families. The population influx from the north was astonishing, to the point that out-of-state license plates nearly equaled those from Texas. While the opportunities were great for these "transplants," adaptation to a different sub-culture and climate, as well as giving up the comfort of family closeness and support, could be stressful. Many adjusted well and embraced a different lifestyle, but others found it too difficult and returned to their native regions.

At the age of twenty-six, Anna took a teaching position in Houston. Patrick, her husband, a chemical engineer, found ample job opportunities for his skills within the "energy capital of the world." Their move from Boston was not an easy one. Anna came from a large Italian family and Patrick from an equally large Irish clan. Both had many siblings, aunts, uncles, and cousins who could not understand why the couple would move away from their families. Sometimes, Anna and Patrick would ask themselves the same when times were tough.

When I first met Anna, she was a healthy thirty-two-year-old and early pregnant. Like many of my new patients during the first few years of my practice, she and Patrick were my age. Some patients viewed my youth as an indication of a newly trained physician, someone up to date with the latest medical knowledge and skills, as well as a peer they could relate to. Others felt disconnected with a "young doctor" who could not possibly have the experience of a mature one. I soon found out that a physician's compassion and conscientious care, and not age, transcend patient doubt and promote confidence. Fortunately, I was able to overcome my novice professional appearance and establish long and trusting relationships with patients who grew up with me.

Anna exemplified the medical phrase "well developed, well nourished female." At five-foot-three-inches tall, Anna weighed 115 pounds calibrated to a body mass index (BMI) of twenty, an appropriate body weight for height. Anna ate healthy, although she would occasionally crave the rich carbohydrate diet of pasta, a food staple from her ethnic background, but exercised regularly and gained only twenty-five pounds during her pregnancy. After she delivered a seven-pound nine-ounce baby boy, Anna was back to her pre-pregnancy weight within four months. The new family thrived well; Patrick was happy with his position with a major oil company, and Anna stayed home to raise Mark.

After six months breast-feeding, Anna went back on oral contraceptives, continued to exercise and eat well, and returned for her routine gynecological exam a year later without complaints. Five months later, Anna was pregnant again and delivered a seven-pound five-ounce healthy baby girl named Joan without complications. Anna breast-fed the second child, exercised and ate well, and lost almost all her pregnancy weight within eight months. Several years later, Patrick underwent a vasectomy, and Anna stopped her birth control pills. She returned to full-time teaching. Few people live storybook lives and Anna was about to face a difficult, and unfortunately, common problem.

Unintentionally, Anna missed her next Pap smear—a result of trying to balance parenting and work. When she came the following year, she looked tired and older than her age of thirty-nine, and twenty-three pounds heavier.

"It's been a tough couple years," she said, more as a statement than an excuse. "You know I've been good about getting my annual exams and taking care of myself, but we had a lot of stress at home," a common response from someone with too much on her plate. Except for Anna, this was literal as well as figurative. No longer did she exercise since her evenings were spent cooking for the family and helping the children with school work. She was also "mom's taxi," driving the kids to their extracurricular activities. Anna claimed, and rightfully so, that she was too tired to exercise even if she had the time. Her eating habits, once healthy, now consisted of quickly prepared meals with limited nutritional value, fatty fast foods, and late night snacking when she tried to "unwind" for sleep and start the process over again. While Patrick helped as much as he could with the family chores, he too was tired and stressed. The couple's scenario was typical for their stage in life, and as I counseled Anna to "try to eat better and get more exercise," I knew, personally, the difficulty in balancing responsibilities with self-care. But I sensed that Anna's words intimated more than the stresses of working and raising a family—and my intuition was correct.

When I asked her if she had anything else to talk about, she began to cry. After regaining her composure, she shared more.

"Patrick lost his job about nine months ago," she said between sniffles. "It's really been tough on him and on our family."

I expressed my concerns. The energy industry took a "nosedive" in the mid-eighties, and Patrick was one of many "casualties." I asked how they were dealing with this additional stress.

"Well," she said with her head turned sideways. "It hasn't been easy. Patrick is quite down and feels bad that he's not the principle bread winner." She smiled. "But things seem more positive. Patrick wants to change careers. He has always wanted to teach, so he's looking into going back to school to obtain a degree in education so he can teach high school chemistry. It won't be easy, but we figure two years of college will do it. We'll just have to get by on my salary."

Changes are always difficult, but career changes are particularly so. It was admirable for Patrick to seek a nobler profession rather than being a pawn in the corporate world. I knew they possessed the strength to make it through this transition. After two years, Patrick finished school and was hired as a high school chemistry teacher in Anna's school district. When Anna came in for her next routine check-up, she looked rested and happier.

"Things are going well," she said with a smile. "Patrick loves teaching and the kids are doing great." She sighed deeply before speaking. "But I'm so frustrated. I can't lose any weight!" Anna gained another seven pounds over the last two years. She shook her head. "I just don't understand it? I'm eating better now, and although I don't exercise as much as I did before, I walk three times a week."

Weight gain is the most common complaint I hear daily. It's a complex issue involving physiologic changes, as well as social and personal influences. Weight results from calories consumed, calories burned, as well as personal genetics. Over fifty percent of Americans are overweight and predictions are higher over the next twenty years. Obesity is a major health problem affecting heart disease, hypertension, stroke, elevated cholesterol, diabetes, gallstones, respiratory dysfunction, as well as a higher risk of death from cancer compared to normal weight individuals. Most profound are the psychological repercussions—poor self-esteem and self-image—and, unfortunately, societal pressures to look thin, as well as discrimination towards obese people, especially in the workplace.

Patients are weighed electively in our office. This option is not based on a blatant disregard, but as a respect for those who find it uncomfortable to share their weight with a nurse or me. Patients concerned about their weight don't need the problem amplified or turned into a "shame and blame" situation. While Anna told me about her weight gain, she declined to be weighed, but her struggles went further, proving to be an additional psychological burden as well.

She gazed at the floor for a few moments before looking at me. "I'm worried that if I don't do anything about my weight now, I'll continue to 'blossom' out of control."

"Why do you think that?" I asked innocently.

Anna stared downward again and I knew there was another worry. She swallowed before speaking. "Both my mom and my older sister are obese. I don't want to become like them," she said fearfully.

Anna didn't explain the psychodynamic differences between her and her mother and sister, but I sensed a lack of approval for their lifestyles or habits. Perhaps this was part of her reason to "move away" both physically and emotionally. While the "Sun Belt" had opportunities, Anna may have viewed her move to Houston as an escape from what she felt was a "no win" environment in Boston. For sure, Anna's fear of obesity was based on many factors, both conscious as well as unconscious.

While there is no "magic bullet" for losing weight, I did take time to discuss dietary changes and the need to find an enjoyable exercise routine sensibly fit for her daily routine. Anna and I talked about options, including weight-reduction programs providing support, encouragement, and an emphasis on the commitment to lifelong changes.

Anna left the office with renewed optimism and determination. She would find time for evening exercise at a local fitness center, an opportunity to work-out without the interruptions and disruptions at home while providing a much needed "time-out" from the burdens of work, children, and domestic responsibilities. Although eating healthier would require changes from Patrick and the children, Anna seemed committed to make changes for her as well as for her family. I knew time would tell if Anna's resolutions were real. Her body mass index was close to twenty-seven, and although she was still in the "overweight" category, I hoped she wouldn't become what she feared the most—obese like her mother and sister.

Five months later, Anna returned to the office for treatment of a bladder infection. While we usually don't weigh patients during a problem visit, Anna asked to be weighed. When I walked into the exam room, she was smiling and proudly asked me to look at her new weight—seventeen pounds lighter.

"Wow," I said with a genuine delight, "you're doing great. How have you done it?"

"Well," she said, "I took your advice, made everyone in the house change their eating habits. I eliminated all junk food including late night snacking. I go to the fitness center five days a week and do weight training, cycling, and yoga." Her eyes were gleaming. "I sleep better and have a whole lot more energy."

I was pleased for her. Anna accomplished something most patients struggle with—she became committed to her resolutions. Anna was not only thinner, but younger in appearance as well. We talked about a target weight for a body mass index of twenty-three, a realistic goal for a forty-three-year-old woman. Her success story was the highlight of my day.

During her next visit, I lifted the chart from the door holder and was surprised that it was almost three years since Anna's last visit. My assumption that she was doing well was erased when I walked into the exam room and saw a heavy forty-six-year-old.

"I know I'm way overdue," she said without making eye contact, "and I'm disgusted with my weight. I guess you just can't change your genes," she said forcing a laugh.

I felt sorry for her, but most alarming was her tone of voice—her resignation for failure. Obviously, the previous commitment to diet and exercise was no longer part of her daily life, but I wondered why she lost her incentives and motivation. I was to find out shortly.

"Patrick was having an affair with another teacher," she said with embarrassment. "I know that may be a lame excuse for my weight gain." She shook her head. "Apparently, it was a short affair, but it still put an enormous strain on our marriage."

I expressed my regrets for an unfortunately common problem, but tried to maintain a professional nonjudgmental role, although I felt anger towards Patrick. I asked what they were doing to make the marriage work.

"Well, we've been going to counseling for quite some time now and it has been helpful. Patrick has opened up about many things, and I can honestly say, I think we have a better relationship now than before."

I was relieved to hear this. Like any other relationship, it takes communication and trust for a friendship to last. While a married couple faces enormous challenges throughout their lives, it requires work to make a relationship healthy. Both Patrick, as well as Anna, had problems that surfaced after they started their family—a typical scenario. Since there are fewer responsibilities when young and newly wed, it's easier for a couple to get along well. But the true test of a solid relationship comes when things are no longer simple, but difficult. The love a couple shares should be the incentive to overcome personal obstacles. Hopefully, Anna's and Patrick's marriage was stronger, but during the emotional chaos, Anna reneged not only on her diet and exercise routine, but found solace in eating, hence her huge weight gain.

"I know I can lose this weight," she said with that recognized determination in her eyes, "but it's going to be harder this time. I'm older and have more weight to lose than ever before."

Anna was correct. It would be an uphill battle, but she had experienced the satisfaction of previous success. With her home life more stable and perhaps less demanding, she could find the discipline she once owned. I knew she had the resolution to commit to a healthier lifestyle, but it would require not only dedication, but a strong inner fortitude.

Anna returned five months later and lost only four pounds in spite of her rigid diet and exercise routine. She appeared frustrated as well as down.

"I'm doing all I can, but I just can't lose it."

I felt bad for her—a common problem for a woman at her age. While I usually don't advocate diet medications, I thought it might help her. There is no pharmacological magic bullet for obesity, but short-term use with strict adherence to diet and regular exercise might provide a jump start for her. Before starting a diet medication, basic blood work is required and the patient must have a body mass index of thirty or twenty-seven in individuals with other risk factors, such as hypertension, diabetes, and elevated cholesterol. Sadly, Anna was now in the obese range.

Two prescription drugs are available, phentermine (Adipex) and sibutramine (Meridia), as well as an over-counter orlistat (Xenical)—all with specific side effects. While phentermine is an inexpensive appetite suppressant, it may cause jitteriness or difficulty sleeping. Sibutramine can cause a dry mouth, weakness, and constipation. Orlistat, a non-systemic medication inhibiting pancreatic enzymes preventing fat absorption from the gastrointestinal tract, can cause increased abdominal bloating and cramps, flatus, and oily spotting from the rectum, as well as a decreased absorption of fat-soluble vitamins, although all can be reduced with the use of daily fiber.

While she seemed reluctant to start a diet medication, Anna felt desperate and agreed to a short-term use of phentermine after obtaining blood work. She was instructed to maintain her present diet, continue with her exercise routine, and return in one month for a weight and blood pressure check.

"I'm going to be realistic about this," she said. "By the way, I've decided to join Weight Watchers. I think the additional support would be helpful."

I was pleased with her reasoning. Anna was not going to be "fooled" by the many commercialized weight reduction schemes. She was too intelligent to fall for these unrealistic fads and gimmicks, no matter how despondent.

Not to my surprise, Anna lost five pounds when she returned for her next visit. "I don't know if it's the medication or Weight Watchers or both, but I feel like I'm on the right track." For some patients, a significant weight loss in the beginning could lead to a "plateau" later. But Anna continued to lose weight. On her next visit, she lost three pounds more, and although she didn't look any thinner, she admitted feeling better, a definite incentive to her commitment.

Anna took the medication for three months and found the Weight Watchers meetings and exercise program more effective. She remained focused on her goal and, although there were constant stresses in her life with the children and work, she did not succumb to comfort foods. She and Patrick seemed to be happy again and, as I hoped, their marriage was apparently stronger. After four months, Anna felt that her weight management visits were no longer necessary, and I agreed.

It took almost eighteen months, but on Anna's next routine exam, her weight had dropped to an extraordinary 131 pounds. She looked and felt great, and recaptured that pretty perkiness I remembered when she was younger. Anna had a new vitality and energy, allowing her to do more as well as dealing with stresses more effectively. Most importantly, she had "out-run" her ghosts—those demons from her unconscious created by her mother's and sister's poor habits. Best of all, she did it the right way, through discipline and determination in a healthy and realistic fashion.

As her doctor, I could only support and reassure, but it took her own motivation and focus to embrace a new lifestyle. Unfortunately, Anna's success is the exception and not the rule. Today's high-paced world and fast foods impede weight management. It was unlikely Anna would ever return to her old habits.

While we all tend to slip into bad habits on occasions, the desire to live a healthier life and feel better is a primal incentive we all possess, requiring recognition as well as commitment. After leaving Anna's room, I took the next patient's chart from the door holder and read the nurse's notes—routine exam, patient complains of weight gain. I took a deep breath and opened the door.

PART VII

# Midlife and Beyond

CHAPTER 14

# Lynn and Vickie

OVER THE NEXT DECADE, a significant number of women will become menopausal. To the year 2010, more than 5,000 women per day, almost 2 million women per year, will turn fifty years old. These baby-boomer women view their gynecological visits as more than a routine examination—a need to check weight, blood pressure, urinalysis, Pap smear, mammogram, bone density testing, fecal occult blood test, as well as lipid and thyroid testing—and the need for counseling about the increased stresses in life and the associated effects on their well being.

Entering menopause produces various physiological, physical, and emotional repercussions. No two women are alike in their clinical manifestations and their reaction, adjustment, and acceptance of these changes. A new controversy has been added to the mix—the concern about hormone replacement therapy—its benefits, side effects, and possible long-term problems. Estrogen, from previous scientific data, was thought to provide numerous advantages, such as the alleviation of debilitating hot flashes, night sweats and vaginal dryness, reduction in heart disease, prevention of osteoporosis, less dental cavities, improvement of skin integrity with less wrinkling, and an overall more "youthful" appearance. But the recent findings of the Women's Health Initiative (WHI) indicated concerns for women taking combined estrogen/progesterone hormone replacement over four years—a slightly higher risk for breast cancer, heart disease, and dementia, while some reduction in colorectal cancer and bone fractures. Recent findings indicate that women taking estrogen without progesterone do not demonstrate an increased risk for breast cancer or heart disease. My preference is for bio-identical hormone replacement—compounded substances made from plants.

105

Although WHI studies have generated criticisms about the methodology used, the findings do raise a red flag and a need to individualize treatment. Hormones as a panacea now require further scrutiny from a scientific perspective. While each patient reacts differently, two of my patients, close friends of each other, presented with strikingly contrasting menopausal symptoms.

A few months after beginning private practice, two personable and talented patients came for their first prenatal visits together, an unusual scenario. An astonishing coincidence had occurred—not only were they early pregnant, but were childhood friends. Growing up in a small East Texas college town, Lynn and Vickie met during their pre-school years. Both girls exhibited creative talents—Lynn was gifted at drawing and Vickie had a naturally beautiful voice. Throughout their elementary, middle school, and high school years, the two best friends developed their inherent aptitudes. Both worked hard at improving the artistic endowments they were given, while blossoming into attractive and amiable young women. Their friendship was so strong that they vowed to attend the same college. Both were accepted to the University of Texas at Austin and the two young women roomed together their freshman year and later as apartment-mates for the remainder of their college life.

After graduation, they each took teaching positions in Austin while continuing to room together, but Lynn and Vickie would not stay together forever. Lynn and her boyfriend Jack decided to get married. Jack was a chemical engineer, found employment in Houston, and he and Lynn moved to their new home after the honeymoon. While no longer roommates, Lynn and Vickie phoned each other almost every day and visited frequently. By coincidence, Vickie's boyfriend, Rex, had become good friends with Jack, and the two enjoyed playing golf together whenever visiting. With one more year left for his pharmacy degree, Rex and Vickie planned to wed after his graduation, although his future employment was still unknown.

Lynn obtained a teaching position in Houston and continued to draw at her in-home studio. She and Jack talked about raising a family, but felt no rush to do so. Each was happy with their career and their new home. But things do have a way of changing for the unexpected.

One evening, Lynn received a phone call from Vickie. Rex found a position in a hospital pharmacy. Lynn was delighted to hear about his good fortune, but Vickie had more to tell Lynn.

"Okay," she said, barely caching her breath. "Now I want to tell you something else that's very exciting!"

"What could be more exciting than what you already told me?" Lynn asked.

"Are you sitting down?"

"What's going on here, Vickie?"

Vickie laughed and blurted out the additional news.

"Rex got a job with a hospital at the Texas Medical Center in Houston! We're moving there next month!"

Both girls giggled and cried at the same time. Neither one ever thought they would be living in the same city together again, but fortune was on their side. Little did they know that a year later, after Vickie and Rex were married and settled in Houston, both would become pregnant with due dates three weeks apart. During their first visit, I learned all about the two's long-term friendship and their unexpected pregnancies. Before they left my office, there was one more bit of information they shared with me.

"Now don't laugh at us," Lynn said with a broad smile. She turned to Vickie who told me the rest.

"We plan to have our babies on the same day," Vickie said as she shook her head excitedly.

I blinked before responding. "Now ladies that would be fine for a story, but your due dates are three weeks apart." I didn't want to burst their bubble, but I needed to be honest and straightforward. Surprisingly, they continued smiling, winked at each other, and left the office with me scratching my chin. How in the world could they be so confident? I shook my head knowing the chance was practically zero. But on each visit, whether together or alone, the subject would be brought up. No, they didn't expect me to induce their labors on the same day, that wouldn't be safe, but somehow, they felt it would happen. It was fun for them to talk about babies with the same birthday, but I was the doctor and I knew best, or so I thought.

Their pregnancies progressed without complications. I enjoyed their visits, especially when their husbands attended, creating an almost party-like scene among the four of them. Both Jack and Rex found it amusing that their wives held to their premonition about the same birth dates, but Lynn and Vickie held on to their improbable belief.

It was early in September when Lynn went into labor. She progressed slowly and, after office hours, I went to check on her condition. She was almost six centimeters dilated, free of pain from an epidural anesthetic. Neither Lynn nor Jack had called either Vickie or Rex to tell them about Lynn's labor. I wrote a progress note in her chart and decided to head home knowing that her delivery wouldn't be for several hours. That's when Vickie and Rex walked in.

At first I thought they heard about Lynn's labor, but I dropped my pen when I saw Vickie stop and grab her abdomen to breathe through a contraction. How could this be happening! But when I examined Vickie, she was five centimeters dilated and in active labor. I pulled my glove off, still in disbelief.

"Vickie, Rex," I said softly. "I, uh, I don't know how to tell you this, but Lynn is in the room next door and laboring as well."

Vickie smiled through her contraction. Jack and Rex met outside the labor rooms and gave each other "high fives." I decided not to go home. I wouldn't miss this for the world.

Lynn delivered a healthy girl at ten while Vickie followed an hour later with a healthy boy. The scene in the recovery room was like a photographic session after a wedding. First, the nurses took photos of the two couples, next with the babies, followed by Lynn and Vickie holding their babies, and finally, with me posing with all of them. The atmosphere was festive and why not? It was fun for everyone, including the nurses. I left the hospital near midnight feeling light and happy. Never underestimate, I told myself, the power of belief.

Lynn and Vickie became excellent mothers, and while they and their husbands remained great friends, their lives took slightly different paths. Lynn was pregnant two years later and delivered another little girl while Vickie had her second child, a girl this time, four years later. With the responsibilities of being parents and maintaining their careers, both women came in for their annual gynecological visits at different times. Lynn opted to undergo a tubal ligation for contraception, but Rex elected to have a vasectomy. It was a delight to see these women at their visits, and always, the subject of that magical night was joyously reminisced. Lynn and Vickie remained best of friends while watching their families grow up together.

Just before turning fifty years old, Lynn came to the office three months before her scheduled routine visit. When I walked into the exam room, she looked tired and pale, a contrast to her appearance during her last visit.

"What can I do for you, Lynn?" I asked, hoping there was no serious physical or emotional issue.

"Doctor," she said. Her voice seemed tensed. "I couldn't wait to see you until my annual exam. I'm miserable! I can't sleep at night because I'm waking up sweating. I feel awful all day—I'm hot and my skin feels like ants are crawling all over it."

When I glanced at her chart, my nurse had noted that Lynn stopped her periods five months before. "Lynn," I asked, "when did the symptoms begin?"

"Well, I've been having them off and on for the past year, but they became real intense about three months ago."

"No periods at all for the last five months?"

"No, not even spotting."

"Any vaginal dryness?"

"Yes," she said staring at the floor, "and Jack and I can't make love because it hurts so much." She looked at me with a desperate stare. "I cry all the time, I'm anxious, and feel down."

Lynn's symptoms were consistent with menopause and her exam revealed pale vaginal walls with tenderness during her Pap smear. I ordered a blood test called a follicle-stimulating hormone, or FSH, a test highly sensitive in differentiating between pre-menopausal and menopausal changes. The next day, the test indicated that Lynn was clearly in the menopausal range.

When she returned for a follow-up visit, I informed her of my clinical impression and the confirming blood test. When I brought up the subject of hormones, Lynn had valid concerns.

"But I've read and heard about the many possible problems with hormone treatment. I don't want to feel this way, but I'm scared to go on them." She swallowed. "I've tried over-the-counter herbal products but they haven't helped."

Lynn was caught in a common dilemma and the latest findings from the Women's Health Initiative added more anxiety to an already stressful life event.

"Lynn," I said, trying not to sound patronizing, "you're feeling terrible and this is not you. I know that taking hormones evokes many different fears, but I truly feel that a woman as healthy as you, one who has maintained her routine exams and mammograms, is an excellent candidate for short-term use of hormones to help you through this transition."

Lynn didn't say anything immediately while she pondered my comment.

"You're right. I'm healthy and fit and my quality of life is more important than the small risk."

Lynn was current on her Pap smear and mammogram. We started her out on a low dose of estrogen/progesterone, a combination hormone necessary since Lynn had her uterus and needed to protect the lining of her womb from overgrowth. She returned for a follow-up visit in four weeks. When I entered the exam room, there sat Lynn the way she used to be—well rested, calm, and cheerful.

"I feel completely different now," she said with a smile. "It took about ten days, but all the hot flashes and night sweats are gone. I feel like my old self again, and the vaginal dryness and pain has lessened. I didn't fully realize how miserable I was just a short time ago."

Lynn continued to do well, and she and I spoke about reducing the dose in about a year and maybe, if Lynn wanted, try and taper off the hormones completely. But for now, she was on the right medication for the right reason.

About ten months after Lynn's initial visit for her menopausal symptoms, Vickie came into the office for her annual exam. There were no complaints listed on the nurse's notes, but I noticed that her last period was six months prior to her visit.

"Vickie," I asked, "do you have any hot flashes or night sweats?"

"No, none at all. And I'm surprised, too. I know what Lynn went through, but I don't feel any different."

Her exam was normal as well. I checked her FSH level and was not expecting the value to be menopausal. But the next day, the test indicated otherwise. I telephoned Vickie.

"While you're menopausal, you don't have any symptoms of hot flashes, night sweats, or vaginal dryness. So I don't recommend hormone use for you. All I ask is that you continue to come for yearly Pap smears and mammograms, take calcium and vitamins, exercise, and have a bone density test with your mammogram next year."

Vickie was comfortable with this management and never experienced anything more significant than occasionally feeling warm. The difference between Lynn and Vickie was a dramatic one. Nothing in their medical or family histories could have predicted such contrasting responses to a similar physiological event. While scientific studies can provide important information for appropriate and wise medical decisions, no one "hat" fits all. Our uniqueness in body and distinctiveness in character is what makes the world a diverse place.

Lynn and Vickie, as well as their families, continued to be close, a testament to their friendship and good values. And while their menopausal responses were different, the night they delivered their firstborns will remain a delightful treat in my memory as well as a mystery of serendipity—or, perhaps, some other unrecognized force.

# CHAPTER 15

# Helen

UNFORTUNATELY, not only are women at risk for cancers that afflict men, such as colon, lung, and brain tumors, but breast, cervical, uterine, and ovarian cancer as well. As a resident, the subspecialty of gynecological oncology interested me, but I wasn't sure if I possessed the emotional fortitude to deal with these diseases. While I try to educate patients on proper nutrition, exercise, smoking cessation, routine Pap smears and mammograms, and appropriate colon testing, it surprises me how many patients do not follow the recommended screening procedures. Sadly, there are those who develop cancer in spite of their conscientious self-care and appropriate medical visits. Such was the case with my patient, Helen.

Although many women worry about ovarian cancer, there is less of a lifetime risk compared to breast or colon. Yet, a good screening test for ovarian cancer doesn't exist. A circulating email purports the need for a woman to have a blood test known as carcinogenic antigen 125, or CA-125. As an advocate for patient health education, I find that most health information on the Internet is correct, but some can be misleading as well as anxiety provoking.

A CA-125 blood test is, however, not a sensitive marker for ovarian cancer screening and is not recommended as a routine test in low-risk women. If a patient is adamant about having the test done, I must counsel her about the potential problems evaluating an elevated value; conversely, a normal value does not confer protection from this cancer either.

Risk factors for ovarian cancer include advancing age, never having children, being of North American or Northern European descent, a personal history of uterine, colon, or breast cancer, or a strong family history for the disease. While still under investigation, fertility drugs do not seem to be associated with an increased risk. Protective factors for women include having a full-term pregnancy and breast-feeding. Surprising to most patients, a hormonal contraceptive, such as the birth control pill, patch, or ring, offers a reduced risk for this disease. By eliminating ovarian activity, the risk of "something going wrong" with ovarian cells is significantly lowered and therefore, a reduction in ovarian disease.

While medical studies have looked at potential screening options—including the CA-125 blood test, pelvic ultrasound, and the combination of the two tests—clinical trial data concludes that a significant number of women would have to be screened in order to detect a few cases. Sadly, these studies showed a minimal improvement in survival even if the disease is detected by a screening methodology. The National Institutes of Health Consensus Conference found no evidence to support the use of these tests except in high-risk women who have two or more relatives with ovarian cancer. For these patients, an annual pelvic examination, CA-125 test, and ultrasound are indicated for screening. Those with strong family history for breast or ovarian cancer are recommended testing for BRCA1 and BRCA2, a blood test to check for specific genetic mutations increasing a woman's risk for these cancers.

A more important reason for cancer screening involves tests for colon, cervical, and breast disease. Sigmoidoscopy every five years or a colonoscopy every ten years is recommended as a cost-effective screening. Unfortunately, about fifty percent of the U.S. population receives colon screening.

The U.S. Preventive Services Task Force recommends mammography for all women over forty years of age every one to two years, although most gynecologists suggest a yearly exam. Nearly one in every ten women will develop breast cancer during her lifetime accounting for approximately 25% of all cancers in women, second only to lung cancer as the leading cause of cancer deaths in women. As all studies indicate, the earlier the detection, the better the chances of a cure.

Invasive cervical cancer should be preventable since the disease has a long pre-invasive state and can be detected by yearly Pap smears. While there exists a rare type of cervical cancer that is hard to detect in a pre-malignant state, most cervical cancers can be detected with advanced technologies used for cytological testing. Additionally, a new vaccine for Human Papilloma Virus (HPV) can confer immunity to many of the high-risk strains that induce cervical cancer. Yet, there are still several thousand deaths from this disease each year in women who do not obtain regular screening.

Surprising to most patients, endometrial cancer is the most common malignancy of the female genital tract in the United States. Higher risk patients, postmenopausal women on unopposed estrogen therapy, obese postmenopausal women, breast cancer patients taking tamoxifen, and those with a family history of uterine, bowel, or ovarian cancer, should be aggressively screened with endometrial biopsies or pelvic ultrasounds. Only fifty percent of women with endometrial cancer demonstrate malignant cells on a Pap smear.

While most patients know me on a physician/patient level, some have chosen me as their doctor after meeting me during a social or professional encounter. As an elementary teacher to my three sons, Helen and I first met at a teacher/parent open house. She possessed all the academic tools—patience, compassion, and a genuine interest in the education of children. My sons adored her kind and easy-going style, and learned well and successfully due to her diligent and dedicated nature. Helen was an impressive person, not only as an educator, but as a parent as well. She and her husband had two children in high school, each an outstanding student as well as athlete. Rob, eldest, excelled at swimming and baseball. His sister, Kim, concentrated her natural athletic ability on volleyball and soccer. Both went on to receive academic as well as athletic college scholarships.

When I first met Helen during a teacher/parent meeting, I noticed a young boy sitting at her desk. He was quiet and well mannered and followed his mother's movements with adoring eyes. Later on, I learned this was Helen's youngest son, Peter, a child born when Helen was forty-one years of age. Peter was a Down's syndrome child.

There exist many myths about Down's children. While they usually have mild to moderate mental retardation, they are easily educated under the right conditions. Some are integrated within regular academic classrooms and partake in most of the social and extra-curricular activities. Many people believe that adults with Down's syndrome are unemployable and incapable of forming close personal relationships. To the contrary, businesses seek young adults with Down's syndrome since they bring great enthusiasm, dedication and, especially, reliability to their jobs. Many Down's adults socialize, date, and have healthy relationships. Perhaps, the myth most misunderstood is their emotional state. Down's children and adults have the same array of feelings as other people, and respond appropriately to positive as well as negative situations and behavior.

Helen came to my office several weeks after our first meeting. Her excellent health paralleled her character. She gave to her own children the same attention she gave to her students. Peter was an active member of his family and loved not only by his parents, but by his siblings as well. He was a happy, well-adjusted child with good self-esteem and a gentle nature. Helen and her family were special people.

Helen never missed an annual visit, obtained yearly mammograms, and underwent a colonoscopy at age fifty. She did not smoke, drank only socially, and exercised daily. Working-out for Helen was like brushing your teeth, showering, and eating, something you did every day no matter how hectic or tired. Her dedication to fitness influenced all three of the children and her devotion to career, family, and her own well being was exemplary. Other than a tendency for a slightly elevated cholesterol level, a family trait, Helen was a healthy fifty-eight-year-old—until the day she came to see me for vague abdominal complaints.

To see Helen other than for a routine exam was the exception. When I walked in the room, she greeted me with her warm smile and looked as healthy as ever. Her last visit was nine months ago—Pap smear, mammogram, bone density, blood pressure, and blood tests all normal.

"Helen, I didn't expect to see you for another few months."

"Me neither," she said cheerfully. "Don't take it personally, but I'd rather not be here!" We both laughed.

"You told my nurse you're having abdominal swelling. Tell me more."

She nodded. "Well, I'm not quite sure what I'm feeling. But for the past three to four weeks, my stomach seems to be protruding."

"Oh," I responded, surprised by her complaint. "Are you having any gastrointestinal problems?"

"No, I'm having regular bowel movements, although I might be having a little bit more gas ... but, no. No real changes."

From her tone of voice, it didn't seem serious. But Helen was not one to complain. Perhaps just an irritable bowel syndrome. Not enough fiber. But I knew Helen ate well and never had symptoms related to her colon.

When I examined Helen's abdomen, there were no unusual physical findings. Good muscle strength was present, although there was a slight "pooch" perfectly consistent with her age, but no tenderness.

"Well, Helen, let's check and make sure there're no gynecological problems here," I said matter-of-factly, not expecting to find anything unusual. But instead of normal uterus and ovaries, her pelvis contained a large pelvic mass, slightly painful to touch. I swallowed.

"Helen," I said as calmly as I could, "I can feel a mass on exam." I was concerned not only about the mass, but the fact that her previous exam was nine months ago.

"What do you think, Doctor?" she asked calmly.

Telling patients what you honestly think is the foundation of a good physician/patient relationship, but the style and manner of communication needs to be individualized, the art of medical practice.

"I'm not quite sure, Helen. We'll order an ultrasound to better define the pelvic organs and a blood test called a CA-125. As you know, the possibilities include a benign ovarian cyst, fibroid tumors, and, not to frighten you, even ovarian cancer."

Helen's countenance changed quickly—a look of concern as well as determination rather than fear. Intuitively, Helen already suspected this worst-case scenario.

"Okay, Doctor," she said without agitation. "Let's do them as soon as possible." Her insightfulness led to the next question. "If we confirm a pelvic mass, and the blood test is elevated, will we then proceed with surgery?"

"Helen," I said softly, "if we suspect ovarian cancer, I will refer you to a gynecological oncologist who will surely recommend an exploratory surgery." I placed my arms across my chest. "Helen, it may be something entirely different."

She smiled again. "Yes, you're right. Let's wait on the test before making any guesses."

Helen left the office cheerful as always. But I knew I'd worry until we had the results.

The ultrasound confirmed a complex mass on the right ovary with both cystic and solid components. More disturbing was the finding of ascites, or fluid in the pelvis, a poor sign suggesting cancer rather than a benign process. I called Helen and gave her the information which she accepted calmly. I referred her to a gynecological oncologist and told her I would call with the CA-125 result as soon as available. As I feared, the blood test was elevated and a CAT-scan ordered by the oncologist confirmed the ultrasound findings but with no evidence of kidney or bowel involvement. Helen was scheduled for surgery the following week. For the first time in her long teaching career, she needed to take time off.

On the day of surgery, I met Helen and her husband in the pre-surgery room. Peter was present as well. At seventeen years of age, he was still well mannered and pleasant and listened attentively to my discussion with his mother and father. When it came time to take Helen to the operating room, he kissed her, told her he loved her, and walked out of the preoperative suite with his father. Just before he left, he turned and said, "Don't worry, Mom. I'll take good care of Dad!" Helen, I, and the nurses all shared a brief moment of levity.

The surgical findings were not good. A pathological frozen section revealed ovarian cancer. But worse, it was everywhere— on her intestines, abdominal cavity, and even on her diaphragm. The ascites, or fluid, was positive for cancer cells. The oncologist and I "de-bulked" as much of the tumor as we could from the pelvis and abdomen knowing that the more cancer we removed the better Helen's chance of responding to chemotherapy. While in the operating room, a surgeon must concentrate fully on the procedure being performed. Sometimes, the doctor chooses music, or even light discussions or jokes to reduce tension. But during Helen's surgery, the oncologist and I operated in almost complete silence for four hours.

We discussed the findings with her family and, as expected, they were attentive and accepted the news without any outward reaction of panic or anger. Their immediate focus was for support. Helen's family was a well-adjusted one, and I knew their energy would focus on Helen's recovery and treatment. But there was one more person involved with this mix—my own self. After the surgery, I remained in a cloudy daze of disbelief and anger. Intellectually, I knew Helen was given appropriate medical care, but ovarian cancer is insidious and usually found late because of its silent nature. Physicians learn to detach in order to be effective as care-providers, but my own emotions at this time were winning out over sensibility, and self-doubt was rampant within my mind.

Helen's clinical presentation was typical for ovarian cancer— no symptoms and no physical findings until the disease is in an advanced state, and even then, the symptoms are non-specific. It took me several days before climbing out of this mental "funk" to refocus on my professional duties. In spite of what the public's perception may be, most doctors are concerned about their patients' welfare and are emotionally disturbed when a patient is ill or not doing well. While some compassion is lost due to the demands and strains of doctoring, most physicians care about their patients.

When I visited Helen on her third postoperative day, she looked well after a long and traumatic surgery and greeted me with her ever-present warm and sincere smile. We talked about what was to come.

"Helen, you realize you'll not be able to teach school for at least six weeks. And that depends on how you tolerate the chemotherapy treatment."

Helen's cheerful countenance changed suddenly. She bowed her head and grabbed a tissue to wipe her teary eyes. Almost instantly, she looked at me with a different expression, one of resolve and determination.

"I don't know what the future holds for me," she said clearly, "but I'm not going to change my dedication to my family, career, or even to my life."

I've never forgotten those words—so simple and yet so emphatic. Sadly, Helen never returned to her beloved role as a teacher. Although she tolerated her chemotherapy well, her illness became worse. Six months after her surgery, Helen became bedridden. The hospice nurses gave her, as well as her family, the necessary support. Her intuition was strong and she never denied or pretended her circumstances. She told her family she wished to die at home in peace and with dignity. Eight months after her diagnosis, she passed away with her husband, three children, and sister at her bedside.

After her funeral, I wrote a letter to the family—a therapeutic catharsis for me and a way to express my sympathy. Helen's husband sent a letter thanking me for my kind words and expressed his appreciation for everyone's care and efforts. What touched me most were his comments on how much Helen valued my compassion and dedication as her physician—words I will cherish forever.

It was several months after Helen's death when I went to our local supermarket to pick up items for dinner. In my checkout lane was Peter, Helen's youngest son, bagging groceries.

"Hi, Peter," I said cheerfully.

At first, he didn't recognize me. Suddenly, he knew who I was and responded with a smile.

"Hello, Doctor! How are you?"

"Fine," I said. "How have you been?"

Peter paused for a moment then lowered his head. Tears welled up in his eyes. Recognizing me as his deceased mother's doctor evoked a strong sense of sadness. But, unexpectedly, Peter raised his head and looked me straight in the eye with an expression similar to his mother's—a look of understanding, acceptance, and resolve. With poise and sincerity, he spoke to me.

"Thank you for taking such good care of my mommy." He turned towards the cashier and began bagging the next customer's groceries with renewed energy.

I don't quite remember what I said to Peter, but I do recall sitting in my car and staring out the window for several minutes before driving away. I needed time to reflect and make sense of everything. It came to me suddenly; while Helen was no longer present on this earth, her spirit was alive and well, and clearly visible on the face of her youngest child, a gifted legacy, powerful and enduring.

# CHAPTER 16

# Betty Jo

EVERY PHYSICIAN, at some time in his or her career, will meet a least one patient who is strange, eccentric, or even just plain bizarre. Only three months into private practice, I recall an interview with a new patient, Pam, a healthy twenty-five-year-old married woman who came in for a routine Pap smear. I noticed she didn't list using any type of contraceptive. My next question seemed logical—"Are you trying to conceive?"

"No, not at all," she said smiling.

"Well," I asked, "do you want to consider anything for birth control?"

"No," she said confidently, "we don't need anything for birth control."

My eyes narrowed. "I guess I don't understand."

"Well," she said nonchalantly, "we don't need contraception because we only have anal intercourse."

While I didn't expect this response, I tried to keep a professional manner, but I wasn't prepared for her next comment.

"That reminds me," she said with concern, "my hemorrhoids have been killing me lately." I stared at her, unable to think of an appropriate reply.

While I've come across some "interesting" patients, none comes close to the uniqueness of Betty Jo. This woman and her husband, Roy, were tough in spirit and rough in appearance after years of farming. The couple managed a low-profit ranch while raising their two kids. They were as different as night and day, but as a couple they created something similar to "folie a deux," a psychiatric condition where two people share the same delusional ideas or fantasies. Although Betty Jo and Roy were not "crazy," their distinctive personalities reinforced each other's eccentricities, producing humorous, and at times, incredulous moments.

While they lived out in the country, the couple came to Houston for their medical care. A primary care physician, Dr. Dave Hunter, referred her to me for evaluation of pelvic pain. Although it is unusual for physicians to call another doctor about a referral, Dr. Hunter felt obligated to warn me. An excellent family physician and well-liked by his patients, Dr. Hunter was a short man, standing at five feet four inches. I was curious why he needed to call me about what seemed to be a typical gynecological referral.

"Listen," he said after explaining Betty Jo's problem, "you need to be prepared for this patient and her husband." Although he was short, his deep resonant voice was commanding.

"What do you mean?" I asked with surprise.

He sighed. "Well, she and her husband are strange, actually, a real trip. Just letting you know, that's all."

I was intrigued. How strange could they be? But I soon forgot about the phone call until the day of their visit.

When I went to meet Betty Jo in the small waiting room outside my office, I saw the older couple reading magazines. At first, they looked like any other husband and wife, except for Roy's overalls and cowboy hat. But when Betty Jo stood up from her chair, her husband did not—or should I say, he couldn't. Roy appeared to be sitting, but actually was standing on a little platform with wheels. As a double amputee, he seemed to be sitting next to his wife. I introduced myself and gestured towards my office. Roy was agile on his platform, moving himself with his hands by pushing on the carpet. Why didn't he use a wheelchair? I thought.

Betty Jo looked older than her fifty-five years of age. Her skin was leathery from years of outdoor sun exposure and she wore no make-up. Her hair, beehive style, appeared comical. Roy was the first to speak.

"Thanks for seeing us, doc," he said with a slow Texas drawl. "The little woman here got her some problem that we just can't seem to figure out what in the world it is." Betty Jo just shook her head in agreement and didn't say a word. I wondered if Roy was going to do all the talking for her.

"No, sir ... can't figure it out. Healthy old gal she is and then 'wham!' she got her this pain in her privates. Now as for me, well, you can tell that I'm as healthy as a horse, except maybe not having no legs or nothing. Lost them things in a accident on the farm years ago. I tried the wheelchair, but it scared the dickens out of my cows, so I found this platform, put some wheels on her, and well, I can get around just as well as if I had four legs!" He let out a big loud laugh. Roy had more gaps in his mouth than teeth.

"Now you take that old Doc Hunter. Really like that Doc," he said with a nod.

"Yes," I replied. "I'm sure you like Dr. Hunter. He's an excellent doctor."

"Naaa, not really," he drawled.

"Oh," I said surprised. I wasn't sure what to say next. But Roy just stared at me like I was supposed to ask him why he liked Dr. Hunter. "Err ... must be his good bedside manner?"

"Well, that he has. But that's not the reason why I like him so much."

I was confused. Why did Roy like Doctor Hunter?

Roy bent towards me and winked. "Well, you see, it's like this. He's the only man I get to talk to when he's standing and be able to look at him eye to eye."

I was about to laugh, but caught myself when I realized that neither Roy nor Betty Jo were smiling. Betty Jo's stare was vapid and expressionless.

I cleared my throat. "Tell me about your problems, Betty Jo."

"Well, you see Doc, it's like this. I woke up a few months ago and had this pain right down here in my lower belly and in my privates that feels like someone stuck a knife in my old belly button, and then twisted it and then kind of turned it into a branding iron that burns my insides like I have never known before. But that was after a night we had some problem with our dogs. You see it's been real dry lately, and you know, them dogs get real spooked if there is thunder, which there was that night ... no wait, was it that night? ... yep, that night was the night my sister called about her old washing machine not working the way it should have. You know, I told her not to buy that kind of washing machine. I said,

'Mabel, that brand just isn't made like it used to be. You need to get you the kind that Roy and I use. Never had any trouble with it.' But that Mabel is as stubborn as our old Papa was and she just do the opposite I tell her just because. You see, Mama didn't like to fight, so Daddy pretty much did what he wanted to and I think Mabel got that from him. Anyways, that's the night the storm came through and the dogs got spooked on account of that. And then the next day, I woke up with this here pain and my neighbor, Clara, thinks I might have pulled a 'groan' or something like that, but what does she know, that woman has no common sense since she got hit by lightning a few years ago and actually lived to talk about. Funny how people can change after them be 'lectrified. Just like that young fella on TV, you know, the one who has those strange people on. You just never know what's going to turn a soul into something that they really weren't, you know, like what was that preacher's name who was on TV and gets thrown in the slammer? Oh, well. Memory isn't as good as it could be. But I'm telling you doc, something is not right with my stomach. And Doc Hunter got me an x-ray that don't show nothing wrong. Well, just ask Roy about that one! Ha!!"

I was lost with Betty Jo's rambling, but I wasn't ready for Roy's contribution to the discussion.

"You know, Doc," he said rubbing his chin. "I looked at that x-ray Doc Hunter got, and I think that x-ray doctor read it wrong."

"What do you mean?" I asked.

Betty Jo chimed in. "Well, you see, Roy know how to read them x-rays because he's half-doctor."

I wasn't quite sure if I heard her correctly. I looked for some sign from their faces, but neither one showed any expression. Did I hear her right? Did Betty Jo really say that her husband was half-doctor, like half-Jewish, half-Italian, or half-Polish?

"You see," Betty Jo said with a blank stare. "Roy is half-doctor. His Daddy was a doctor, so he knows these kinds of things."

I think my jaw fell open. Roy nodded in agreement with his wife. They were serious and convinced that he possessed inheritable physician skills from his father. I swallowed hard. Dave

Hunter was right—there was something mystifying about this couple. Once I regained my composure, I tried to obtain more information from Betty Jo about her previous gynecological history and surgeries as well as her symptoms, including gastrointestinal and urological problems. But with every answer she commented about her cousins, dogs, children, grandchildren, crops, weather, vacations, and sundry unrelated events. We were twenty minutes into the history before I realized the interviewing was going nowhere. I dreaded to ask the next question, but I knew I had to. Yet, looking at Roy sitting on his homemade platform, I wasn't sure how to approach it. I needed to know if Betty Jo experienced dyspareunia, or pain during intercourse, but I wasn't sure if the two engaged in sexual relations. I formulated my question in a way I thought was diplomatic.

"Betty Jo," I asked. "Are you sexually active?"

She twisted her lips and frowned. Now I felt bad. Either Betty Jo was too embarrassed to admit it or Roy was ashamed about his compromised manhood, but I was learning that nothing was quite what I thought it might be with this couple. Betty Jo's insipid stare seemed like an eternity before she responded.

"Well," she said, "I do get up on top sometimes."

My eyes widened in disbelief. I wet my lips before speaking. "Uh, let's go to the exam room and see what we find." Maybe, I thought, a change of venue would help. I gestured towards the exam room and asked Betty Jo to slip off her dress and put the sheet across her lap. I needed a break from Betty Jo and Roy. I went to the kitchen, gulped down a diet drink, and tried to regain focus. Please, I thought, let the exam go without any further incidents. I was an hour behind with office patients, but had a hunch more surprises were in store.

When I walked in, Betty Jo was sitting on the exam table with the sheet across her lap as instructed. I asked her to lie back and put her feet in the stirrups so I could examine her. I sat down on a stool, put lubricant on the speculum, and turned towards her pelvis only to abruptly stop the exam when I noticed Betty Jo's pantyhose between me and her vagina. I shook my head.

"Uh, Betty Jo ... I can't examine you with your pantyhose on," I said as calmly as I could.

"Well," she said. "I thought you were going to have some problems. Why didn't you tell me to take them off? You just told me to slip my dress off only."

"You're, you're right," I said incredulously. "Why don't you take off your pantyhose and I'll be right back in."

I couldn't believe it. What in the world did she think I meant? Quickly, I went in to see another patient while Betty Jo changed.

I returned again and asked her to lie back and put her feet in the stirrups. This time, when I rolled my stool over to start the exam again, there was another obstacle between her pelvis and me.

"Betty Jo," I said trying to restrain my annoyance. "You need to remove your panties before I can exam you."

She sat up quickly. "Well, I thought so, but you didn't tell me to," she said angrily. "I kept thinking that maybe you did it some other way."

I sighed. "No. No, there is no other way," I said exasperated.

When I returned for the third time, Betty Jo sat on the table completely naked. Her white pendulous breast contrasted with her sun-damaged neck.

"Uh, we're not going to do a breast exam today," I said.

"I know, you told me that before, but I thought that you're probably having a bad day, since you haven't explained real well to me what to take off and so forth, so I decided not to take any chances and help you out by going naked."

My nurse swallowed her laugh as I sat on the exam stool, dumbfounded and dismayed.

"Thank you," I said, but my voice was weak and soft. I wasn't sure how to handle Betty Jo. Her perplexing personality made me feel inept. Finally, I was able to exam her. Other than generalized tenderness throughout the pelvis, there was no indication of any uterine or ovarian masses.

After she dressed, I spoke with Betty Jo and Roy once again and offered her further imaging studies or a diagnostic lapa-roscope to rule out pelvic pathology such as endometriosis, a generalized inflammatory condition of the pelvis. They stared at me, faces blank, before Betty Jo made one more strange comment.

"Well, I bet I know how I got this condition."

"Betty Jo," I said. "I'm not completely sure that you have endometriosis, but only a suspicion. And besides, if you do have endometriosis, we really don't know how one gets this condition."

"Doc, I know what you're saying, but I don't think you're right."

I tightened my lips. "What do you mean?" I said trying to prepare myself for another twisted explanation.

She turned towards her husband. "Roy, do you remember when we took the grandkids to Disney World a few months ago?"

"Sure I do," he said with his wet gums glistening. He turned towards me. "Best fun we've had in years."

"Well, we may have had fun, but that's where I caught this here disease," she said while nodding her head.

What did her gynecologic complaints have to do with Disney World?

"Yep ... that's got to be it. Cause I think some of this here pains started after that vacation."

"Betty Jo," I said in disbelief. "Why do you think you caught endometriosis at Disney World?"

She smiled at me like I was some first-year medical student who didn't quite grasp clinical medicine yet. "Doc, where else would you get 'endo-mickey-osis' at, but at Disney World?"

My eyes widened.

"You know, old girl," Roy said. "I bet you're right. Being half-doctor, I should have knowed that!"

I don't remember the rest of Betty Jo's visit, but I know I spent the rest of day catching up on the schedule and trying, albeit unsuccessfully, to put Betty Jo and Roy out of my mind.

A few days later, my nurse told me that Betty Jo called and scheduled a laparoscope and that she hoped I would be more on the ball than I was in the office. I rubbed my tired forehead, hoping I would be ready for her hospital admission. But during her preoperative visit, she and Roy seemed sensible and focused. They even agreed to a hysterectomy if endometriosis was discovered and found untreatable by medical therapy. Maybe it was me that was "off" during her first visit.

On the day of surgery, I talked to Betty Jo and Roy in the preop room and went over the game plan. Surprisingly, neither one said anything odd. Once anesthetized, I looked into Betty Jo's pelvis with the laparoscope and saw that her uterus, tubes, and ovaries were riddled with endometriosis along with significant adhesions surrounding her intestines and bladder. She needed a hysterectomy. The surgery was long, tedious, and physically draining. After several hours, I put the final stitch to her incision.

Betty Jo did well the first day of surgery, but developed a fever and some nausea the next day. An abdominal x-ray confirmed my clinical suspicions—Betty Jo had an ileus, or a physiological slowing of the intestinal function, a common result from the extensive surgery. Treatment includes IV fluids while the gastrointestinal tract is put at rest by prohibiting food or drink. Usually, twenty-four to forty-eight hours resolves the condition. When I explained my plans to Betty Jo, she gave me her trademark expressionless stare.

"I don't understand, Doc," she said. "I don't understand why I can't eat?"

"If you eat something too soon," I said while patting her leg, "your intestines will stay like they are and you might get sicker. I can't feed you until you pass gas." I knew she didn't agree with me, but I hope she understood why.

Her condition was unchanged the next day, and again, she asked why she couldn't eat, requiring me to explain the process and treatment again. After office hours, I telephoned her nurse who informed me that Betty Jo was stable but had not passed gas yet. I was surprised she wasn't better, but hoped the ileus would resolve by the next day. But at around nine that evening, I received a page from the hospital. Betty Jo's nurse was frantic.

"We can't find her anywhere!"

My eyes narrowed. "What? How long has she been missing?"

"Since seven this evening. I had security check all over the hospital."

Where was she I thought? "Was her husband with her?"

"Yes, and he's gone too!"

What were they up to? Quickly, I grabbed my coat and left for the hospital. Did she go home when I wouldn't feed her? I started to get anxious—one of my patients was lost and with a post-operative complication to boot. I hurried through the corridors racking my brain about what to do. Call the police? Call her children? But when I arrived on the hospital floor, the nurse shook her head and told me they were back in her room. She and her husband decided that not eating couldn't be right, so they left the hospital, he on his platform and she in her opened hospital gown while pushing an IV pole, and walked to a local supermarket about ten minutes away. When I entered her room, Betty Jo was finishing a ham sandwich while Roy was eating a "Moon Pie" and washing it down with a beer.

"Doc," she said with a serious look. "You know, you're a decent fella and Roy and I like you. You did a good job with your knife on me. But sometimes, I don't think you have a lot of common sense."

I stared at her, trying to prepare for their logic.

"How in the world can you fart if you don't have nothing in your gut?" she said with squinted eyes. "So, me and Roy decided to take matters in our own hands, and although that store had the sorriest tomatoes I have ever eaten, I bought the meat, bread, lettuce, and mayo and made this here sandwich. Roy picked up a snack for hisself since this hospital has the poorest food, and no ice chest for beer." Roy nodded as he took another swig.

"Now, you see, Doc," she said as if she was a full-time faculty professor at a medical school, "I ate this sandwich, a poor excuse for one if you ask me, but I ate it anyhow, and it wasn't just five minutes after that I started to fart real good." Roy just shook his head in agreement.

Stupefied by her explanation, I examined her abdomen, now soft and flat. When I listened with my stethoscope, amazingly, her bowel sounds were active, her ileus resolved.

"Well, Doc?" she asked. "How does my belly sound?"

I swallowed. "Uh, good, Betty Jo. I think you're all better."

She raised her chin. "Like I said, Doc, you can't fart unless you eat. Don't they teach you that kind of stuff in doctor school?"

"Uh, yes, yes Betty Jo." I was lost for words. Roy chimed in.

"When will we get the old gal home?"

"Probably tomorrow," I said softly.

"Better go and get some sleep, Doc," she said admonishingly. "You look tired."

I nodded, turned, and left the room, but before I closed the door, I heard a loud and sonorous explosion of flatus coming from Betty Jo's bed, followed by Roy's deep belly laugh.

"You sound like the horses do, you ole gal you!" he shouted. Betty Jo was laughing uncontrollably and passing loud flatus at the same time.

She did go home the next day. Two weeks later, she returned to the office and was doing well. At six weeks, I examined her again and found her fit to return to normal activity. But the Betty Jo and Roy act had an encore and now I was part of the skit.

"Doc," she asked, "can I get back on my tractor?"

"Yes, I see no problem," I answered.

"Well, can Roy and I have sex again?" she asked.

I don't know what came over me, but I lost some of my professionalism and answered her question in an uncharacteristic way.

"Betty Jo," I said smirking, "not only can you get on your tractor, and not only can you have sex, but you can have sex while on your tractor!"

I couldn't believe I said this! While there are times I may retort with something witty or earthy, this was not my style. Both Betty Jo and Roy stared at me with their usual expressionless faces. I wanted to retract what I said. Obviously, they didn't find it humorous, and I feared that I insulted them. But, as in the past, I was wrong.

Betty Jo turned and looked at Roy before making eye contact with me.

"Hmmm," she said reflectively. Roy was rubbing his chin pensively.

"You know, Roy," she said. "The Doc's right. Might save us some time."

I shook my head in disbelief. Betty Jo and Roy thanked me again, although I wasn't quite sure if it was for the medical care or for the last comment. I still see Betty Jo and Roy every year. Her visits are low maintenance since she no longer has her female organs. I never brought the subject up about my off-color comment. But, every time I leave the room, Roy looks up at me with his almost toothless grin—and winks.

# CHAPTER 17

# Greta

ONE OF THE MANY BURDENS of a gynecologic practice is the daily routine and the repetitive complaints: weight gain, decreased libido, mood changes, tiredness, depression/anxiety, and the various vaginal infections. While each patient's problems are unique and must be addressed with professionalism and compassion, a doctor and his staff sometimes feel like the proverbial "broken record" discussing the same issues *ad nauseam*. Yet, there are those patients who deal with the enormity of their problems so courageously that they make all other complaints seem insignificant and foolish. Such was the case with Greta.

Born and raised in Germany, the seventeen-year-old Greta met Hans, a twenty-year-old American soldier, after WWII. Greta's daughter, Rita, a patient of mine, told me that her parents' photographs from their early married years revealed a happy couple—she, a pretty and vivacious young woman, and he, a remarkably handsome and dashing young man. Hans was a native Texan, a first generation American from German emigrant parents who came to the United States and settled in Fredericksburg, Texas, a quaint town in the Texas hill country. Hans spoke German fluently and played minor-league baseball in the Texas League before being drafted into the army. Greta learned English quickly, and after their marriage, the couple moved to Texas, where she worked with her husband raising cattle on a ranch outside Hans' hometown. While he no longer played baseball, Hans' passion for the national pastime was fulfilled by coaching little league teams, a difficult task considering the demands of ranching.

Greta worked hard to help run the ranch, and together, they raised two children, a boy and a girl. When Hans turned sixty-five, they sold the ranch and moved to Houston to be close to their two children and four grandchildren. At her first visit, Greta appeared to be an extremely healthy sixty-two year-old with a bubbly personality who spoke articulately with a slight Germanic accent interspersed with Texas colloquialisms such as "y'all" and "fixin." She and her husband bought a small home near their daughter's family and enjoyed their retirement years. Without missing a step, Hans became involved in youth baseball as a coach, and he and Greta went to almost every game, watching the youngsters improve their baseball skills. For many years, Greta's annual visits were a refreshing respite from the quotidian burdens of practice, a mixture of medical care and lively conversations about the game of baseball, my passion as well. When my three sons played in the same youth league, Greta and I talked about the fields, the games, and, of course, the enjoyment of the sport.

One day, she came to the office for treatment of a bladder infection. After talking about the youth baseball league and the number of "rain out" games during a particularly wet spring, I asked Greta if everything was going well. That's when I learned about a family problem.

"Well," she said slowly and with a hint of sadness. "You know how things can change so quickly." This was an unusual departure from her optimistic personality. "My seven-year-old grandson was diagnosed with leukemia four months ago."

"Oh, I'm so sorry to hear that, Greta," I said with sincere concern. "How's he doing?"

That's when her most infectious smile appeared and the ebullient personality resurfaced. "Oh, he's doing very well!" she said with enthusiasm. "He's a strong little boy and hopefully will be in remission soon."

Greta left the office with that unique brand of delight that my office staff was used to. Later that day, when I thought about how I would react if one of my children had been diagnosed with cancer, I shook my head to get the morbid thought out of my mind. Greta's acceptance of life's vicissitudes and her upbeat attitude were courageous and inspiring. But there was to be more pain in her life.

On her next visit, Greta, who had always looked healthy, came in using a cane to help her ambulate.

"What happened to you?" I inquired with genuine concern.

"Oh, it's really nothing," she said casually. "I broke my leg a few months ago at a baseball game. Silly me! I slipped when trying to leave the bleachers and fell off the top bench!"

"Greta, I'm so sorry!"

"Oh, no big thing. I'm getting around much better now," she said with a big smile.

I was afraid to ask, but felt I needed to. "How's your grandson?"

"Well, he did go into remission, but now the doctors are a little bit concerned about a possible recurrence. But he looks great and is playing baseball again this season. We'll find out next week about his tests," she said smiling. I swallowed hard. Could nothing bring this woman down?

On her next visit, Greta still walked with a cane. Her leg fracture had not healed as well as her orthopedist hoped, and Greta would occasionally experience a shooting pain in her leg as well as difficulty walking.

"I keep talking to my leg to get better," she said grinning. "But the darn thing is about as stubborn as my husband Hans!"

Again, I cautiously approached the subject of her grandson.

"Oh, he's doing great now. The blood tests did show a recurrence of the leukemia and he underwent some more chemotherapy. Poor Carl, he had so many side effects from the drugs. But he's doing well and is in remission again, thank goodness!"

But there was more, and Greta's face became serious. She spoke slowly and calmly.

"While Carl was getting his chemotherapy, Hans had a heart attack."

My eyes widened. "Is he okay?" I asked nervously.

"The old fool," she said with that special smile. "He's doing well after a coronary by-pass and is coaching again!"

I was relieved. Not only was Greta strong, but her family was as well—supporting one another was the key to their resiliency. Greta left the office while sharing pleasantries with the staff. Her presence brought a lighter spirit to the office atmosphere and made the rest of the day more tolerable.

Greta returned a year later, now using a walker to ambulate. While her skin still appeared smooth and youthful, her eyes looked old and tired. I hesitated briefly before asking about her family. Greta didn't smile and stared downward. I knew something was wrong.

"Carl's doing very well," she said softly. She looked at me with tears gently rolling down her cheeks. "Hans passed away a few months ago." I swallowed hard and wet my lips. Greta wiped her eyes and regained her composure. "He was doing well, but one night, while at a baseball game, he felt funny. He thought he was just tired, but he never woke up."

My heart hurt for Greta. She and Hans had been married for almost forty-eight years. How does one recover from such a loss? A faint smile came across her face.

"You know, the funeral was very beautiful. The kids asked the minister to do something different during the ceremony, something that was very special to me," she said. "They played 'Take Me Out to the Ballgame' during the service. The whole congregation sang." She shook her head. "Hans would have been very happy."

The large lump in my throat made it difficult to speak. Somehow, Greta and I got through the visit, although my heart remained heavy for days. I found an appropriate sympathy card and mailed it. A week later, I received a package from her that contained a small framed quotation that remains on my desk ever since:

"Duty makes us do things well, but love makes us do them better."

Now I knew part of the secret for Greta's strength.

Greta returned a year later, but now wheelchair bound under the guidance of her daughter. Her usual upbeat personality remained in spite of her condition. She talked about baseball, her children and grandchildren, and how well Carl was doing. Then I learned something new.

"Doctor," she said with her eyes focused and clear. "I had surgery a few months ago, but I'm coming along well."

Not another traumatic event I thought.

"Yes, well you see, I fell again, but this time I had a seizure. When my family took me to the hospital, they discovered a brain tumor on the x-rays. It was cancerous, but I'm tolerating my radiation treatments well."

Again, I was shocked. What this woman had experienced over the last several years was more than most would see in a lifetime. And yet, her personality did not change. She remained cheerful, optimistic, and appreciative for everyone's help and support. If only I could develop just a fraction of this woman's strength and courage, I would be a better person. But that was Greta—unflappable in her belief for the best, as well as her refusal to become depressed, cynical, or angry. I thanked her profusely for her inspirational gift and she left the office in her usual way with smiles to all the staff.

I never saw Greta again. I learned of her death from her daughter, Rita, who came in for a routine exam and told me that her mother had passed away from the brain cancer.

"She was happy till the moment she died," her daughter said, wiping away her tears. "The grandkids loved her so much. It was just as hard on them as it was on my brother and me."

"Duty makes us do things well, but love makes us do them better" remains on my desk and Greta's inspiring and courageous personality is felt whenever I read the message. And every time I hear "Take Me Out to the Ballgame" during the seventh-inning stretch, I feel the strong and special presence of Hans and Greta.

# PART VII
# Physicians

## CHAPTER 18

# Dr. Meyers

Every day, phone messages come across my desk—sometimes from other physicians, personal acquaintances, and people who are trying to sell me something. But, on occasion, I'll get a message from an attorney asking if I will consider reviewing a medical liability case or perhaps act as an expert witness. The world of jurisprudence is a complex one, especially concerning medical-legal issues. While I find nothing edifying about the legal process, it is a necessary part of our societal rules and regulations to help maintain law and order.

Although I have little interest in participating as an expert witness in a medical-legal lawsuit, there are cases which I feel a moral and ethical responsibility to become part of—the circus of documents, depositions, mediation, and possible trial proceedings. While I do little expert witness work, I believe in being cordial and professional. Every message from a lawyer will get a return call, although most cases presented to me, either by the plaintiff or the defense attorney, seem frivolous and unjustified. However, one phone message intrigued me, involving another physician whom I had met during my residency training.

Dr. Joseph Meyers was an older obstetrician-gynecologist who performed deliveries and surgeries at one of the teaching hospitals I rotated through during my postgraduate years. A man now in his early seventies, Dr. Meyers was your quintessential physician—proper in speech, impeccably dressed, courteous and cordial to all the staff. While I worked little with him during my training, I would, on occasion, have an opportunity to talk with him in the doctors' lounge, usually between two and five in the morning. His manners were faultless and his patients were devoted to him because of years of excellent care. No matter what time of the day, Dr. Meyers would walk into the male doctors' locker room wearing his trademark bow tie, and would calmly change while meticulously hanging his clothes in a locker. When getting ready to leave the hospital, he dressed slowly, and would comb his hair and straighten his bow tie to perfection before stepping back into the hospital corridors.

His gentlemanly ways were impressive and he was always calm, even when things were hectic. After having assisted another staff physician with a cesarean section at five o'clock one morning, I went into the doctors' lounge for a cup of coffee to help start a day that never ended the night before. There was Dr. Meyers, sitting in a chair and reading a medical journal. He looked up at me.

"Good morning!" he said cheerfully. "Looks like you have had a busy night."

"Yes," I said, my voice tired and hoarse. "Things haven't stopped for a minute ... three cesareans, two ectopic pregnancies, and three ER admissions." Our rotations through the private hospitals were usually tame, unlike the two county hospitals, but this particular night was not.

"Well, well," he said softly. "At least you're getting excellent training. I'm sure you'll sleep well tonight."

If I make it through the rest of the day, I thought. But Dr. Meyers' soothing voice did bring me down a notch, and I felt calmer.

"Dr. Meyers," I said. "I assume you're waiting to birth a baby?"

His eyes brightened and a smile came across his face. "Yes!" he said excitedly. This is the mother's fourth baby, and I'm proud to say I have delivered all of her children."

His fatherly presence was cherished by his patients and why not? He had all the time in the world when it came to taking care of them, and unlike most of the other obstetricians, Dr. Meyers, amazingly, took his own call except for an occasional brief and needed vacation time. Most of the staff obstetricians found this strange, but Dr. Meyers felt that he was the one chosen by the patient, and therefore, obligated to deliver her baby.

Although exhausted, I decided to sit and converse with him. "How many years have you been in practice, Dr. Meyers?"

"Almost forty years," he said proudly.

I sipped on my coffee. "How do you take your own call every day and every night without any breaks?"

He paused for a moment and rubbed his chin as if he never thought about this question before. "Well," he said quietly. "It's like this. Every time I deliver a baby, I just light up like a Christmas tree!"

I looked at Dr. Meyers for a few moments before saying anything else. The genuineness and joy for his beloved patients and profession was real and unselfish. He was someone special—an actual version of an idealized physician—a rare breed. But I also learned from other staff doctors that his life had not been without tragedy. Dr. Meyers had two children. His daughter was a nurse and worked in the medical ICU at the hospital, but his son's life had taken another course. While in high school, Ryan was constantly in trouble with disciplinary problems. He managed to graduate, but went from one odd job to another. At nineteen, he was drafted into the army and sent to Vietnam. After being there for two weeks, his patrol was ambushed by hidden Vietcong and the entire patrol was killed except for Ryan. Dr. Meyers left his practice for three weeks to be with his son at an army hospital in Japan. After multiple surgeries, and with his father by his side, Ryan succumbed to his injuries. A few years later, Dr. Meyer's wife died, and again, he took several weeks off. The staff doctors said that when he returned to work, despite the grief, his perfect manners and pleasant personality were unchanged.

When I returned the attorney's phone call, she told me that Dr. Meyers was named in a lawsuit and asked whether I would consider reviewing the case and possibly becoming an expert witness. The law firm representing him obtained my name from another doctor who did legal work for them. I didn't ask for any particulars, but I couldn't fathom who would sue this humane doctor. Happily I agreed to review the case.

About a week later, I received a large envelope containing papers about the lawsuit. I needed time to sit and read all the documents carefully—the plaintiff's attorney's subpoena, the patient's medical records, and the depositions of Dr. Meyers and the plaintiff. I waited for an opportunity to read the information without interruptions; but when I found time one Sunday afternoon, I read accusations that enraged and saddened me at the same time.

Mrs. H, a long-time patient of Dr. Meyers, was diagnosed with metastatic breast cancer. Dr. Meyers was her obstetrician/gynecologist for over twenty-five years and delivered her three children. According to the subpoena, the patient alleged that Dr. Meyers should have made the diagnosis earlier before the cancer had spread to her spine and lungs. While missed breast cancer diagnosis is a common reason for medical liability suits, it can be a difficult disease to detect for certain types of malignancies and is not always found by standard radiographic techniques. In most cases, routine mammography has given doctors the advantage of diagnosing the disease years before the patient or the physician palpates a malignant tumor. Usually, the reasons for the suits are based on a negative mammogram in spite of a tumor present, or the doctor not pursuing further studies when a patient presents with a breast mass. Knowing Dr. Meyers' thoroughness, I assumed the cancer wasn't detected by the mammogram and that Dr. Meyers was named in the suit along with the radiologist and the hospital.

But when I went through the legal documents to see if there were other defendants, I found that Dr. Meyers was the only one listed. What happened with Dr. Meyers and this patient? Further reading told the whole story.

According to his deposition, Dr. Meyers saw the patient yearly for well-woman exams, and repeatedly suggested she obtain a routine mammogram, but she refused to do so. Further on in the deposition readings, I learned that the patient told Dr. Meyers she would rather die from cancer before finding out if she had the disease, and that no women in her family ever developed breast cancer since they usually died from heart disease instead. It was only after she came to his office with a breast lump that she agreed to obtain a mammogram. After the cancer was diagnosed,

Mrs. H's oncologist told her that it might have been cured if found earlier by mammography, but now the prognosis was significantly lowered.

While Mrs. H admitted she didn't obtain a mammogram, she insisted that Dr. Meyers didn't emphasize the importance of mammography, and she would have done it if he was more meticulous about her well-woman care. Dr. Meyers came from an older generation of doctors who wrote a limited amount of information on a patient's office chart. While my contemporaries have been taught to document all details, Dr. Meyers felt his time was more worthwhile when spent attending to the patient rather than working on a piece of paper. His office chart did not indicate a recommendation for mammography, although it was unlikely Dr. Meyers wouldn't stress the importance of this test. While his records were brief, I knew better about his professional diligence and conscientious care. I was sympathetic towards this patient and her bout with cancer, but I was angry that she would blame Dr. Meyers for her own irresponsibility and immaturity; even more so, I was livid that an attorney would accept a meritless case.

I read the legal documents twice, taking notes, and drafted a letter to the defense attorney stating my position: Dr. Meyers had not committed malpractice and had provided appropriate care to Mrs. H. in a way that was in accordance with the standards of proper medical conduct. Surely, I thought, this case was going nowhere, and hopefully, it would be dismissed. But I was wrong.

After all the appropriate legal issues were obtained from the plaintiff as well as the defense attorney, the case went to mediation. While I didn't attend this meeting that included the two lawyers, as well as Dr. Meyers and Mrs. H., I found out later that the mediation was unproductive towards a resolution. While Mrs. H. and her attorney put the entire blame for the patient's missed breast cancer diagnosis and her subsequent medical bills, mental anguish, and loss of wages on Dr. Meyers, he was as adamant about his proper and correct medical care. Neither party would compromise—Mrs. H. for emotional reasons and Dr. Meyers for his belief that he did nothing wrong. Now the case was scheduled for trial by jury.

For doctors, the medical legal world is a foreign environment where the laws of the land take precedence over the laws of medical theory and logic. When I came to the courthouse to give my expert witness testimony, I saw Dr. Meyers sitting next to his attorney, wearing his traditional bow tie. As I answered questions, first from the plaintiff attorney followed by the defense lawyer, I could see, from the corner of my eyes, Dr. Meyers nodding his head in approval as if my presentation was for academic morning rounds. After my testimony, I listened with indignation as the plaintiff's expert witness gave his interpretation. The doctor was part of a physicians' group despised by most of my colleagues—"hired guns" or physicians who testify against other doctors for monetary incentives. His comments and criticisms were unfounded and unjustified. Dr. Meyers kept his head slightly bent and never demonstrated any umbrage, his self-restraint uncompromised. I left the courthouse in a rage. Surely, the jury would see through all this and acquit Dr. Meyers.

A few days later, I received a call from the defense attorney. I sat in disbelief when she told me about the guilty verdict against Dr. Meyers.

"The plaintiff's attorney was a real wordsmith," she said. "And he befuddled and confused the doctor while he was on the witness stand. I guess the jury looked at him as an old man who should not be practicing medicine. That, and their sympathy for Mrs. H's guarded prognosis, must have convinced them that he was negligent and so they found him guilty."

I fell back into my office chair and stared out the window. It was ludicrous for decisions to be made by jurors without medical knowledge or logic. The current system is wrong, unfair, and needs reform. Suddenly, I felt a deep compassion for Dr. Meyers—a man who dedicated his life to caring for his patients and now a victim of an unjust legal system.

Several months later, I interviewed a new patient and found out more about Dr. Meyers. She told me she had to find another doctor because her previous one had retired. My eyes narrowed when I asked her who the doctor was, although I sensed what her reply would be.

"Dr. Joseph Meyers. You know," she said after sighing, "he was my doctor forever. I just loved the man. He delivered my children, performed a hysterectomy on me several years ago, and also took care of my two daughters. I was shocked to hear about his retirement. A wonderful doctor ... as well as a wonderful person. I'm going to miss him."

I checked with some of my colleagues who worked at Dr. Meyers' hospital, and found out that he indeed closed his practice a few weeks after the trial. Not surprisingly, he took the outcome hard and I assumed his confidence was shaken. No one had seen or heard from him in months.

About a year later, I was attending a continuing medical education conference when I saw Dr. Meyers sitting at a table dressed in his finest suit and wearing his famous bow tie.

"Glad to see you!" he said with enthusiasm while shaking my hand. He looked dapper and healthy. I expressed my disappointment about the outcome of the trial and he politely thanked me for my support.

"You know," he said with some reflection, "I became quite down after that. I couldn't sleep, lost my appetite, and didn't want to see anyone. Then a few months later, I realized that I missed practicing medicine and that I was a good doctor. Why should I let a little setback like that stop me from doing what I love? So, I now work at a community clinic three days a week and enjoy doing it. I get to help those in need who appreciate my care, and best of all," his face revealing a big grin, "I get to sleep all night long!"

I smiled with him—for his newfound passion, for his emotional fortitude, and most of all, for his uncompromising dedication to his profession.

CHAPTER 19

# Dr. Raymond

WHILE MUCH EMPHASIS is placed on the physician/patient relationship, there is another interaction within the medical profession requiring understanding, compassion, empathy, and support—the physician/physician relationship. Although the roles are different for the doctor and patient, communication and camaraderie between physicians is complicated by personalities who are usually focused, driven, and, at times, egocentric. While most physicians respect their colleagues, there are some who are detached, supercilious, territorial, and selfish. Most physicians are friendly and cordial with their peers, but others are distant and adversarial.

Such was the case with Dr. George Raymond, an obstetrician/ gynecologist who came to our hospital a few years after I began practice. While respected by the nurses for his clinical knowledge and skills, Dr. Raymond remained aloof with most of the medical staff, and later, even more so with me. When I first met him, I received a "cold shoulder." One of my colleagues gave me the inside scoop.

"The guy never smiles or talks to anyone. He doesn't share call, and when he goes out of town, he pays someone to cover him rather than to reciprocate. Stay away from him. He's a jerk and then some."

Why is he so antisocial with his colleagues? I thought. "Does he have a family or any friends?" I asked.

"No, he doesn't. Everyone assumes he's divorced. Who could live with someone like that?"

It seemed tragic for this man to live his life this way: alienated, and perhaps, miserable. I wasn't about to pass judgment on him, or at least not until I had the chance to understand him better if the opportunity presented itself. But my colleague seemed to have pegged him well—Dr. George Raymond had few words to say to anyone on the medical staff. When he came to department or hospital meetings, he'd sit by himself. I would always say "hi" to him if we passed in the hall, but he rarely made eye contact, and if he did, he wouldn't speak or gesture a response. Surprisingly, I never heard nurses complain about his bedside manner or ill-behavior towards them. He kept to himself for whatever reason, and rather than become angered by his actions, I accepted his choice to remain unfriendly.

While it is common for patients to request their records when transferring to a new doctor in another city or for insurance purposes, a request for records to another colleague can create bad feelings. Today, with managed health care dictating their rules, it's not unusual to receive a record request when a patient has a change in her health provider. While most doctors claim that a record request doesn't bother them, in truth, it is a figurative slap in the face and a major ego buster. Intellectually, it is far better for an unhappy or problem patient to seek her care somewhere else when the art of medicine is compromised, but I never thought a record request would upset a physician as much as it did Dr. Raymond.

A new patient came to my office for her first prenatal visit and a request was made for her previous records. While her medical history was uneventful, I was interested in reviewing her chart for completeness, not knowing that Dr. Raymond was her previous obstetrician until I received a phone call from him a week later.

"Look," he said loudly, "it's bad enough that we have more doctors on staff than this hospital needs, but then you steal one of my patients. I'll never forgive you for this."

I was flabbergasted. This was the patient's choice, not his nor mine. I tried to maintain my composure.

"If this ever happens again, I'll report you to the medical staff and to the local medical society for unethical behavior!"

He hung up before I could respond and tell him that it was he who was way off-base and unprofessional. I shook my head in amazement and decided it was not worth my energy to let him get under my skin. It was his problem, not mine. But, still his reaction was unsettling. I took pride in my ability to get along with patients, nurses, and especially, other physicians. Yet, Dr. Raymond's rage was inappropriate and personally, as well as professionally, insulting.

Fortunately, for the next several weeks, our paths did not cross. While I knew he was wrong, I felt a twinge of anxiety meeting him at the hospital. Perhaps, I thought, he might even apologize for his outrage, claiming a "bad day" as an excuse. But my assumption was wrong. As I came out of the doctors' lunch room one day, there was Dr. Raymond. This time, he made eye contact, but with an angry scowl. His gaze was so intense that for a moment I thought he might take a swing at me, but he turned his head straight ahead and walked on. His acrimony wasn't normal.

When Dr. Raymond's previous patient came for her next prenatal visit, I felt a need to find out why she changed doctors, curious if Dr. Raymond's polemic personality was the cause. Surprisingly, she liked his care and thought highly of him and changed only because a friend of hers was my patient. If she found Dr. Raymond rude, uncaring, or difficult to understand, I could accept his reaction towards me. What made him so livid? Perhaps, when the timing was right, I could confront the conflict on diplomatic terms, and hopefully, resolve the issue with him, but I didn't expect the opportunity to occur so soon and under such difficult circumstances.

It was around 5:30 one morning when I laid my head down in the doctors' lounge, having been awake since three AM attending a laboring patient. Her delivery was difficult, but the outcome was good—an eight pounds, five ounces healthy baby boy. I hoped to sleep for an hour before showering and heading to the office for morning clinic. Instantly, I fell asleep, only to be awakened ten minutes later by loud knocking on the door.

"Doctor," she yelled, "we need you in the OR 3 stat!"

Feeling disoriented, I jumped from the bed and tried to regain my focus. Was something wrong with my patient? I rushed towards the operating room wearing my surgical hat and shoes and with a surgical mask tied to my neck. The light in the OR suite was blinding, but my vision cleared quickly when I entered the room.

I'll never forget the look on his face. Dr. Raymond's eyes told it all—intense fear. The anesthesiologist was squeezing an IV bag into a catheter trying to push more fluid into a patient. Blood was everywhere—the drapes, floor, Dr. Raymond, and the scrub nurse. Dr. Raymond spoke with a shaky voice.

"Ruptured uterus! Big blood loss! I need help!"

The patient's uterus had ruptured, or split, at the previous cesarean scar. Later, I learned that the patient was awakened by severe, stabbing abdominal pain with vaginal bleeding. Fortunately, she lived only ten minutes from the hospital. The husband wisely called Dr. Raymond's answering service before they left. Once notified, Dr. Raymond headed for the hospital immediately.

The blood loss was extraordinary, so much so that her bleeding vessels spewed red tinged watery fluid instead of the usual deep red. Quickly, I helped Dr. Raymond find the uterine vessels and begin an emergency hysterectomy. The anesthesiologist panicked when he couldn't get a blood pressure or pulse.

"I need blood now or we're going to lose her," he yelled at the circulating nurse.

"Please don't die," Dr. Raymond whispered softly. "Please don't die."

While working in silence, we completed the surgery after two hours. Fortunately, the patient survived, and, miraculously, came through without permanent damage. When I left the OR, Dr. Raymond said nothing further. I was tired and emotionally drained but confused as well, not because of our lack of communication, but for the human side Dr. Raymond revealed under the ordeal of the emergency. Surely, I thought, the man must have some kindness within him.

A few days later, I received a phone call from Dr. Raymond. While not particularly friendly, he expressed appreciation for my help and that he wanted to "repay" me for my assistance by inviting my wife and me for dinner at his house. I paused, not sure how to respond. Yet, I was intrigued and wondered if this was the opportunity I was seeking—a chance to understand this complex man. After conferring with my wife, I accepted his invitation.

His modest one story home was decorated with interesting paintings and sculptures. Dr. Raymond lived by himself and seemed comfortable in his own environment. While he seemed more at ease, I still felt a tension between us. He was cordial and friendly to my wife as they made small talk about his artwork. His articulate discussions about each work of art as well as the artist were enlightening. As the evening progressed, I learned more about his interests.

He was a wine connoisseur and selected an outstanding bottle, complimenting the flavorful hors d'oeuvres, discovering that he was a gourmet cook as well. Not surprisingly, he seemed to relax as the evening progressed. I saw a different side to this man, the antithesis of his reputation among the staff doctors. Now I was even more curious. Why the Jekyll and Hyde personality? I was to learn soon.

After dinner, we went into his living room for coffee and dessert and we continued our lively conversations. Dr. Raymond's angry façade faded as his personable, intelligent, and generous side was exposed. When it was time to leave, we thanked him sincerely for a wonderful evening of good food, conversation, and enlightenment. Before we left, my wife noticed a photograph of an attractive woman holding an infant.

"What a beautiful photo. Is that your sister and her baby?" my wife asked innocently. He swallowed hard and stared at the photo before responding.

"No," he whispered. "That ..." He paused. "That's a photo of my wife and baby girl." His eyes were misty. "I, well," he said and paused again. "They died in a house fire many years ago," he said softly.

We were shocked—an awful tragedy. He seemed to regain his composure. He wet his lips before speaking.

"Well, I haven't talked to anyone about it much, except for Kim's parents who still live in Florida. I'm an only child and both my parents died many years ago." He sighed. "I was in Labor and Delivery that night. Kim loved candles and fell asleep while feeding the baby, and, well ..." His voice faded into silence. He nodded. "I had to get away from Florida, so I moved away to start a new practice."

What do you say to someone still grieving? My wife and I expressed our sympathy.

"You know, this was good for me, tonight," he said. It's the first time I've actually felt alive since I moved here." He shook my hand. "Please, let's do it again. And, thanks for helping me that night in the OR ... I would have lost the patient without your help."

Dr. Raymond did change after that night, but it took time. Slowly, he became friendlier with his colleagues. His sorrow and anger wore heavy on him, but he realized it made things worse. It took that evening for him to open up and begin to heal. After another year, he was a different person—pleasant, cordial, and friendly, with many talents and interests. He asked to join my call group for weekend coverage and vacation time, and he volunteered to be on several hospital committees, contributing time and input. My wife and I became good friends with him, going to museums and eating at restaurants he selected for their special cuisine; and whenever our paths crossed, a strong and friendly handshake replaced an angry stare.

PART IX

# Conclusion

# CHAPTER 20

# Medicine and
# the Human Condition

As STATED IN THE INTRODUCTION, these "clinical tales" are composites of many different patients and circumstances, reflecting
the human condition. Perhaps the great American poet, William
Carlos Williams, also a dedicated physician, wrote best about this
theme in his essay entitled, "The Practice" that appeared in his
autobiography.

> It's the humdrum, day-in, day-out, everyday work that is the real
> satisfaction of the practice of medicine. [T]he actual calling on peo-
> ple, at all times and under all conditions, the coming to grips with
> the intimate conditions of their lives, when they were born, when
> they were dying, watching them get well when they were ill, has
> always absorbed me.

The burdens of medical practice are numerous: from the strain
of listening to patients and their complaints; the need to maintain
adequate continuing medical education in an ever-changing field;
the threat from medical-legal liability; the difficulty maintaining
an economically successful practice due to constraints from managed health care; the tense skills and concentration required for
surgical expertise; and the physically and mentally draining hours
tending to patients' diseases and their associated emotional states;
but it is the trust a patient puts into his or her doctor, a reward
without equal, that transcends these onuses.

This humanistic approach to medicine has been introduced,
on a limited basis, in medical school curriculums. While a small
part of medical education, it is a necessary requirement. Reading

excerpts from literary works with medical themes enlightens, and more importantly, mitigates the technological overload medical students are exposed to. How refreshing it is to read stories, poems, or essays dealing with themes such as the perspective of the patient, the education and responsibilities of a physician, the emotional burdens other colleagues have experienced, and the affirmation that the discipline of medicine is an art as well as a science. Students relate to these topics, as well as emotionally purging their anxieties and fears, permitting them to redefine their focus for the nobility of medicine. Hopefully, medical school curriculums will expand their use of medical humanities to include art, theatre, and writing as well as literature, a means to promote empathy, professionalism, and self-introspection.

All the stories in this book reflect a universality that is part of the human spirit—the hope to maintain good health and the fear of illness and death. This common denominator overcomes social, cultural, racial, ethnic, and religious distinctions. Although illness is perceived differently, the primal emotions remain human. Medicine is a discipline within an area of scientific knowledge that is limitless. As practitioners of this art, physicians learn to combine their medical knowledge with the ability to communicate compassionately. To heal requires more than a good bedside manner, but faith and acceptance, as well as courage and strength by both parties—the physician and the patient.

As previously stated, there are many purposes to this collection of vignettes—to inform, to edify, to intrigue, and to be touched by this universal spirit that we all share—the innocence of Amy and the bravery of Jessica; the confusion of adolescence as depicted in the stories about Carrie and Cindy; the obstetrical challenges of Laura and Alice; and the repercussions of naivete demonstrated by Sarah and the twins, Janet and Lisa. Other topics include the topic of obesity as presented in the story about Anna, and the differences in menopausal symptoms and treatment as seen with Lynn and Vickie. Part of this mix includes surgical complications as revealed in the story about Cathy; the survival of domestic violence depicted in the chapter about Lucy; the anguish of divorce experienced by Jill; the unconventional patient as revealed through the story about Betty Jo and her husband; as well as the courage of living and dying with cancer as read in the vignettes about Helen and Greta; and the complexities of the physician/physician relationship as demonstrated by the stories about Drs. Meyers and Raymond.

While these stories are about women, the themes are not gender specific. Every male knows a female intimately, bringing them into the arena of women's health. Dr. M. Scott Peck, author of the sage book, *The Road Less Travelled,* wrote: "Life is difficult. This is the great truth, one of the greatest truths—it is a great truth because once we see this truth, we transcend it."

Such is the substance of these stories—the human drama—a journey of joys, tragedies, and affirmations for the gift of life.

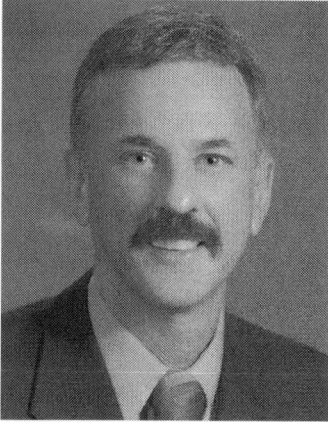

# About the Author

RANDY BIRKEN was born in 1950 and received a B.A. cum laude from Adelphi University in 1972 and a medical degree from Boston University in 1976. He completed his residency in Obstetrics and Gynecology at Baylor College of Medicine while serving as chief resident in 1980. Board certified in 1982 and re-certified in 1995, he is a fellow of the American College of Obstetricians and Gynecologists as well as the American College of Surgeons. In addition to his private practice in gynecology, uro-gynecology, and laparoscopic pelvic surgery, he is an Assistant Clinical Professor of Obstetrics and Gynecology at Baylor College of Medicine.

In 1997, Dr. Birken enrolled as a graduate student at Houston Baptist University and completed his Master in Liberal Arts degree in August of 2000. He has taught undergraduate literature as well as lecturing to medical students on literature with medical themes.

Medical publications have appeared in the *Journal of Obstetrics and Gynecology, Ob-Gyn News, Obstetrics and Gynecology,* and the *Journal of Reproductive Medicine.* Dr. Birken has published a short story in the "Internal Milieu" section of the *Archives of Internal Medicine,* a poem entitled "In a Candle's Flame" within a collection entitled *The Wounded Heart,* an essay in the *Journal of Graduate Liberal Studies* entitled "Painted Poetry: Charles Demuth's Visual Interpretation of William Carlos Williams' 'The Great Figure'," and a short story in the 2004 issue of *Dermanities* entitled "Court Room Medicine: Without a Pulse or Conscience."

He has completed a collection of clinical vignettes as well as a novel. *A Harvard Death and Other Stories* was published by Blue Dolphin Publishing in 2006 and *Her Longest Marathon* in 2008.

In addition to his love for literature, teaching, and writing, he is an avid cyclist, fitness enthusiast, golfer, baseball aficionado, pianist, and amateur radio operator. Dr. Birken has three sons, four step-children, and three granddaughters. He and his wife, Liz, live in The Woodlands, Texas.